Financing Dental Care: An Economic Analysis

Financing Dental Care: An Economic Analysis

Paul J. Feldstein
Professor
University of Michigan

Lexington Books
D.C. Heath and Company
Lexington, Massachusetts
Toronto   London

Library of Congress Cataloging in Publication Data

Feldstein, Paul J.
  Financing dental care: an economic analysis.

  Bibliography: p.
  1. Dental economics.   2. Dental care- United States- Statistics. I. Title.
RK58.F4   338.4'3   73-1013
ISBN 0-669-86181-2

Published simultaneously in Canada.

Printed in the United States of America.

International Standard Book Number: 0-669-86181-2

Library of Congress Catalog Card Number: 73-1013

To My Parents

Contents

List of Tables

Table

Table

Table

List of Figures

Preface

This study was initiated when Dr. William Brown, Dean of the School of Dentistry, University of Oklahoma, asked me to write a relatively short paper on "Funding and Payment for Dental Care." Due in part to my lack of knowledge on the subject this rather lengthy manuscript evolved.

The book is intended for those persons interested in the financing and provision of health services. For this group, which includes more than health economists, I have included explanations (hopefully sufficient) to minimize the reader's need for a technical background. Economic concepts have been explained whenever used; the tools of economic analysis are discussed and illustrated; and technical aspects, which underly various observations in the text and which should be of interest to economists and health professionals, have been placed in appendixes.

I especially wish to thank Owen MacBride for his helpful assistance, which has greatly facilitated this project. Ralph E. Berry and Jeremiah J. German read an earlier draft, and I am grateful to them for their many helpful suggestions. I have also benefitted from the comments of Alex Maurizi and James Jeffers. Needless to say, I am responsible for the errors remaining. Ann Webster has done most of the typing for me and I wish to thank her for her patience.

This work was supported by US Public Health Service grant number HS 00041.

Financing Dental Care: An Economic Analysis

1

Introduction — Needs in Dental Health Care

This book will not provide specific answers to any of the important questions regarding the financing of dental care. Instead, its purpose is to attempt to make explicit the choices involved under alternative financing schemes. The decisions on the mixture of financing arrangements and the magnitudes of each are, and will continue to be, based upon a complex set of political, social, and economic factors. The role of the economist, therefore, is to provide information on the choices available and the costs and benefits of those choices, so that the public and their representatives can make better choices.

The necessity to make choices presumes a situation where there is scarcity; and problems of scarcity are the concern of economists. When considering the question of financing dental care, it becomes obvious that there are not (nor is it likely that there will be) sufficient government funds to finance all the dental programs that some persons would desire. Therefore, we are faced with a problem of how to make choices, given limited government funds, to achieve certain desired goals.

Before discussing objectives and financial desires in the field of dental care, it is perhaps useful to place the "needs" in dental care in perspective with relation to other needs, and to consider the competition between these needs for scarce government funds.

It would be difficult to find a group of professionals who did not agree that there are a great many unmet needs in the population they serve. This observation has proved especially true with respect to health services but it would probably be equally true in any identifiable group of providers. However, solutions to the problem of what to do with such unmet needs would generally meet with less unanimity. Usually, at least in the health field, the designation of unmet needs is coupled with a recommendation for funds to provide resources and to pay for care to eliminate such needs from the population. Such recommendations regarding how to meet such unmet needs (professionally defined) are affected by considerations such as the effect of increased supplies of manpower on the professionals themselves (perhaps in terms of their incomes), the method used for reimbursing the provider, for delivering such care, and so forth.

Every profession must believe that the unmet needs of the population they serve are more important to the well-being of society than those of other professions. An outsider to the dental profession, in addition to being less informed, is also likely to be less biased as to the relative value of various unmet needs among professions.

1

The funds required to provide for all our unmet needs would be staggering. In every area of social concern — e.g., health, education, welfare, housing, the environment, as well as in matters of national defense, transportation, etc. — the sums requested, if granted, would greatly exceed the funds available or the amounts that taxpayers would be willing to spend.

The question, then, is how do we as a society choose from among all these requests for unmet needs. Complicating this decision process is the problem that it must be a *continual* set of choices: for as funds are allocated to one set of priorities, additional available funds should probably be allocated to a different set of priorities, because the *relative* size and value of remaining unmet needs has changed.

The Economics of "Optimal" Oral Health Status

Economics provides a framework within which the questions of financing may be viewed. Within this framework, alternatives can be posed and the relevant data can be suggested for research in order to cost out these alternatives. The numerous value judgments present in any subject on financing should also be made explicit so that it becomes possible to estimate the costs of different value judgments — and, once a value judgment is adopted, to determine the most efficient way of achieving it.

If we as a society were today to spend all that is required to insure that there were no further unmet dental needs and that "optimal" oral health (as defined by the dental profession) were achieved by all, what would be the "cost" implied by this choice? In order to describe the costs of such alternative choices and to specify the necessary data and research requirements involved, reference is made to Figure 1.1, which shows the relationship between oral health status and the alternative ways in which these dental expenditures can be funded, e.g., on programs for increasing manpower, research, etc.[a]

A second empirical question is where on this curve are we currently? If we are closer to the bottom, then for a given increase in dental health expenditures a large increase in oral health will be achieved. If we are already spending a great deal of funds on all such programs we may be near the top of the line where only minor increases in oral health will occur with continued increased expenditures. Although there may be an absolute increase in oral health status with increased dental expenditures, the increase in oral health status with such

---

[a]For simplicity we have skipped a step; instead of relating expenditures on a program to the increase in its output and then describing the relationship between increased output from each program (more dental graduates) to oral health status, we have omitted this intermediate step and just discussed the relationship between increased expenditures on a program and its effect on health status. For decision making, this intermediate step is important if we are to have more accurate information on the expenditure-oral health relationship. This is another empirical question for which research is required.

additional expenditures will be smaller than previously; that is, there are decreasing marginal returns. Similarly, we must ask the same question with respect to each of the dental programs which we propose to fund. Depending on the program and on how much has already been spent on that program, some programs will bring about greater or lesser changes in oral health status than others.

To further simplify the discussion, we have omitted certain effects that are important and which are research questions: Namely, an increase in expenditures on a particular program may, in addition to moving along that program's oral health status curve, cause shifts in the relationship between other programs and their oral health status curve. This would occur where these programs are complementary or substitutable to the one being funded. For example, increased expenditures on fluoridated water will cause decreases in the number of caries while increasing the return to those programs that attempt to decrease peridontal diseases.

To summarize the discussion up to this point, in order to make choices with respect to expenditures on oral health we need to know:

1. What are the alternative programs that will increase oral health status?
2. What is the relationship between oral health status and increased expenditures on each of these programs?
3. What is the overall relationship between oral health status and increased expenditures on dental health (merely summing up the relationships for each program)?
4. At what point are we currently on the curves for each program?

There are two policy questions for which we would use this information, if it were available. The first is, given a limited amount of funds, how should they be spent so as to result in the largest possible increase in oral health status? The criteria to use in order to answer this question is to spend the dollars so that the *change in oral health status per dollar spent in each program is equal.* In other words, continued expenditures on some programs will bring about smaller increases in oral health than other programs because of decreasing marginal returns to any one program. The assumption that with continued expenditures on a program the return from that program begins to diminish is implicit in the curve shown in Figure 1-1. Therefore the way to spend those funds most efficiently is to spend the funds on those programs where the change in oral health is greatest per dollar spent. (Since it costs unequal amounts to increase the output from any one program, this is adjusted by dividing the increase in oral health achieved by that program by what it costs to achieve it. Those with the highest return per dollar should receive the greatest amount of funds.)

This method of allocation suggests that those programs which are currently the largest shouldn't always receive the most funds. It also suggests that a continued evaluation of the return to each program must be made, and that it is

Figure 1-1. The Relationship Between Dental Health Expenditures and Oral Health Status

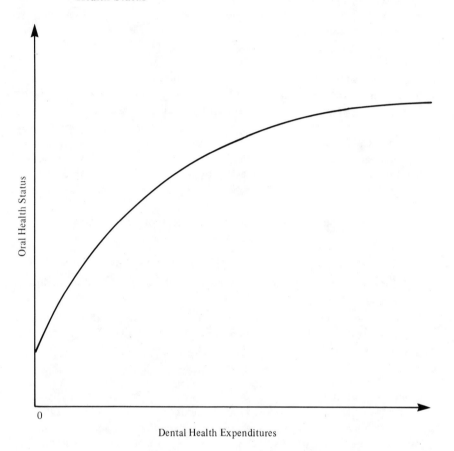

Dental Health Expenditures

important to know the relationship between the output of that program and expenditures on it.

The "cost" of continued expenditures on any one program, therefore, is the effect on oral health status that could have been achieved had those dollars been spent on other programs; the true "cost" of meeting all the needs in any one area are the unmet needs that could have been met in other areas.

Second, how much should be spent on dental health? To achieve a level of financing in the area of dental health that would virtually end all unmet need for dental care would probably be a poor allocation of society's scarce funds. Such an approach would require society to be in a position far out on the curve between dental health expenditures and oral health status. Continued increases in oral health would only come from large additional expenditures (because of decreasing marginal returns). Meanwhile, other societal needs would still be at the lower part of their curves. For in order to move along the dental health expenditure curve, we would have to move backward along the curves of other needs. As wealthy a society as we are, we still could not be at the far end of the curve with respect to all our needs. Where we end up on the dental health expenditure curve depends not only upon the values we place on meeting various needs but also upon the cost of doing so.

If the dental profession is to increase its share of federal and state funding for its various financing programs, then it must be able to determine the effects of such increased expenditures. Further, it must be able to set priorities among programs in terms of the cost of achieving a change in oral health status. To date we have virtually no information on these relationships, not only for dental health but also for health services and most of the government financed human resources programs.

The Specification of Objectives in Oral Health and Their Implications for Financing Strategies

Specifying an objective, e.g., increasing the oral health status of the population, is a necessary first step if we are to be able to list the alternative methods that can achieve that objective. Too often legislative objectives are specified that are really subobjectives — for example, increasing dental manpower — which then preclude from consideration widely varying alternatives that may have a higher return to increasing oral health status than does a particular program.

There are two basic objectives in the dental health field. The first and perhaps the more important is an "equity" objective. An equity objective implies a redistribution of income from those with higher incomes to those with lower incomes. It thus involves a series of value judgments, such as whether or not lower income persons should be subsidized by those with higher incomes, and if so, by how much, under what conditions and mechanisms, etc. When applied to oral health (or dental services) this income redistribution objective implies that, based on a value judgment that some people are not receiving as much dental care as some persons believe they should, a policy decision is made to improve the oral health (or to increase the use of dental services) of a particular population group.

This redistribution goal can be implemented in a number of ways: The government could finance the demand for such services (a national dental insurance plan), or it could finance an increase in the supply of dental services. Under both these government financing programs, the use of dental care will be increased. How good a redistribution policy each of these alternatives are depends upon which income group benefits most in relation to their contribution to the financing costs of the program.

There are a number of value judgments involved in income redistribution policies and these will be discussed separately later. We discuss the income redistribution objective in order to suggest that all government programs that have this objective (although probably not stated in this way) should be considered as alternatives to each other and compared to see which ones most directly achieve their objectives: the redistribution of dental care to those with lowest incomes by financing the programs from those who can most afford it. That is basically the criteria to be employed when evaluating any income redistribution program.

Within any such program there are differing values as to how much dental care should be redistributed. These values will be made explicit in the analyses that follow so that we can determine the most efficient way of achieving a given set of values. In this manner we hope to separate the areas of controversy in financing dental care into differences in values and empirical differences, i.e., the magnitudes and effects of different programs. Most of the existing and proposed financing programs in dental care are income redistribution policies that range from increasing the demand for dental care to increasing the supply of such care.

The other major objective of concern is economic efficiency. This objective raises several questions: How well does the market for dental services perform? Are there market imperfections (restrictions or externalities) that cause the level of dental services to be lower than it would be if such restrictions were removed and the relevant social benefits and costs were included? (Chapter 6 contains a more extensive discussion of economic efficiency and the "optimal" level of output.)

Since these two broad objectives are rarely articulated, it becomes difficult to evaluate specific financing programs and suggest alternatives. For example, if a market does not perform adequately because there are restrictions that result in higher prices and lower quantities, this does not suggest that there should be a financing program to deal specifically with this problem. It may instead mean that a nonfinancing program would be preferred. Unless the dental sector is evaluated in light of these objectives it is not possible to prescribe the relevant policies, whether they are financing programs or otherwise.

Programs once established have a life of their own. Special interests are developed that make it difficult to change either the direction or the magnitude of funds going to such programs. As we have discussed above, continuing evaluation of all programs is required if scarce funds are to be shifted to those areas with the greatest need. Therefore, in light of the two objectives — income redistribution and efficiency — questions will be raised and comments made regarding various traditional policies and alternatives to them. Hopefully, a clarification of issues and values will result.

An Economic Model of the Dental Care Sector

Following is an economic model of the dental care sector showing how the various parts interrelate so that it becomes possible to evaluate alternative policies, in different parts of the model, with regard to a common objective. Examples using introductory tools of economics are developed that will introduce those readers without any background in economics to the concepts that will be employed in later chapters and will indicate how a more complete model of the dental sector can be constructed based upon the separate markets for dental services, dental manpower, and dental training facilities.

There are a number of reasons why it is important to have a clear concept of the dental care sector when considering the financing of dental care. Foremost is the need to have a common understanding of the interrelationships of the various parts of the sector. In this way it is possible to trace the effects of any changes in one part of the sector throughout the system. Such a model can be used for forecasting; for example, what will be the effect of an increase in the number of children in the population on the following: the demand for visits, the price of a visit, total expenditures on dental care, the demand for dentists and, ultimately, on the number of applicants to dental schools. The forecasting example might also work the other way: How would an increase in the supply of dentists and dental auxiliaries affect the number of visits supplied?

Additional uses of such a model naturally flow from the conceptualizing of how the various parts are interrelated, as well as our ability to forecast the effects of any changes throughout the system. For example, if we are considering one program for government financing of dental care, then such financing could be undertaken at different parts of the dental sector. We can finance the demand for dental care or, alternatively, subsidize dental students. Only by having a complete model of the dental sector is it possible to see that these might be substitute strategies in achieving a common goal. It might, as well, allow us to compare their effects on the basis of per dollars spent in each program.

A schematic diagram of the dental care sector would be useful at this point to describe each of these purposes in greater detail and to indicate the kinds of data to be collected and the type of research needed if we are to make better choices among existing and proposed government programs.

Figure 1-2 describes, in a broad sense, the various levels in the dental care sector. At the highest level we are concerned with the demand for and supply of oral health.[b] By this we mean the demand and not just need, since what is needed may not be translated into demand. Economists are concerned with understanding and forecasting demand rather than need. By understanding the determinants of demand it is possible to suggest policies that would translate need into demand, if desired. Further, unless planning and forecasting are based

---

[b]In a broader sense we should be concerned with the overall level of health, in which oral health is just one part, together with physical and mental well-being. In this context we are again faced with the same kinds of choices when we discuss alternative ways of achieving "good" oral health — that is, if our goal is to increase the level of health status, what is the relative contribution, at any point in time and among different population groups, of achieving higher levels of oral health at the "cost" (the foregone opportunity) of spending those same scarce resources on the other inputs to health status. In competing for government funds to improve oral health, therefore, the dental profession must be able to justify such an allocation in light of this broader goal. For purposes of this discussion, however, we take as given the desired objective of improving dental health and examine alternative strategies within this subobjective.

8

Figure 1-2. A Model of the Dental Care Sector

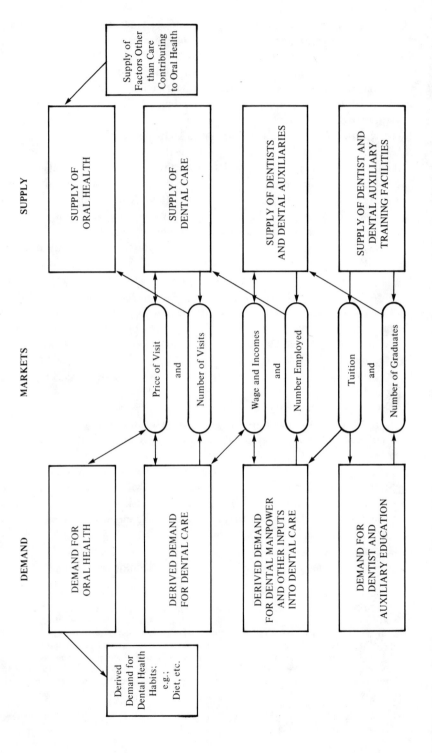

on demand rather than need, we will end up with surpluses and excess capacity if the need is more than the amount demanded.

The demand for oral health and the demand for dental care are not necessarily synonymous and they have therefore been separated. Persons interested in "good" oral health will have a demand for a number of factors contributing to oral health, such as certain foods in their diets, various appliances used in the care of their teeth, as well as for good dental care. The demand for dental care (care produced in a dentist's office) is therefore a demand derived from the initial demand for "good" oral health. It is important to separate these two demands for more than semantic reasons. If the real policy objective is to raise the level of oral health in society, then there are various alternative methods by which to achieve this goal. One might be to subsidize (hence increase) the demand for dental care. Other alternatives might be to affect the demand and supply of other factors contributing to good oral health, e.g., fluoridating water supplies. The policy selected will depend on a number of factors to be discussed, among which are the relative costs of implementing each program and their effects on the presumed objective, the level of oral health.

Although the emphasis in this book will be on dental care, it is important to keep in mind that dental care is only one way of increasing the community's level of oral health, and that at some point there might be better returns (in terms of increased oral health) from financing programs other than dental care affecting oral health.

The determinants of demand at each of the levels specified in the model described in Figure 1-2 are the results of a number of factors to be discussed in more detail later. Suffice it to say that unless these determinants are specified and the magnitudes of their effects ascertained at each level, it will not be possible either to forecast accurately nor to evaluate the effects of different policies.

Returning to the model, then, there is a demand for dental care which is derived from a demand for good oral health. From the interaction of the demand and the supply of dental care, which consists of dentists, dental auxiliaries, capital, and equipment, are determined the price and quantity of dental care. The determination of, and changes in, price and quantity are the subject of economic analysis. The familiar terms "supply and demand" are the economist's classification system for analyzing price and quantity. An analysis of *both* supply and demand is required in order to predict what price and quantity will be. For example, a study that uses demand alone and attempts to forecast future dental utilization without considering supply may be seriously in error. Similarly, any attempt to forecast dental prices without discussing demand will also be inaccurate.

This can be seen more readily with reference to Figure 1-3, which is a hypothetical diagram of the supply and demand for dental care. Since it is two-dimensional, it only shows the relationship between the price of dental care and the quantity of dental care. The line D (representing demand) is the

Figure 1-3. The Demand and Supply for Personal Dental Care

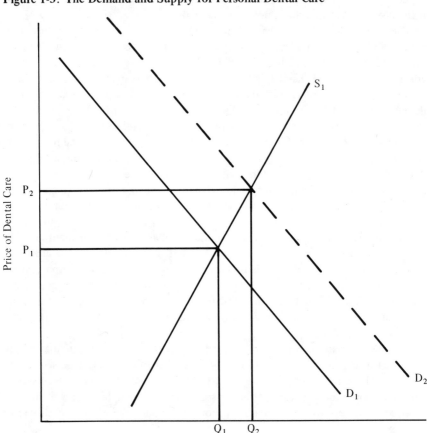

Quantity of Dental Care per Year

relationship describing the quantity of dental care people would buy at different prices; at lower prices more will be bought. (Other factors affecting demand are not shown, other than to indicate where the level of demand is on the quantity axis.) The supply curve shows the increased amount that would be supplied at higher prices — again, other factors being held constant.

The intersection of demand and supply (D and S) determines the Price (P) and Quantity (Q). If one of the factors affecting demand were to increase, e.g., attitudes toward seeking dental care, then this would represent a shift to the right in the demand curve which would now be D_2. Under this situation, if supply were unchanged, we would forecast increased prices (from P_1 to P_2) and increased utilization (from Q_1 to Q_2). Expenditures would also increase (from $(P_1 \cdot Q_1$ to $P_2 \cdot Q_2)$, or the area represented by the new prices and quantities. If, however, the conditions of supply were such that instead of looking like S, it were more like S_2 in Figure 1-4, then with an increase in demand, price would be lower and quantity greater (P_3 instead of P_2, and Q_3 instead of Q_2), and total expenditures also less ($P_3 \cdot Q_3$ instead of $P_2 \cdot Q_2$). A knowledge of supply and what is likely to happen to it becomes crucial in forecasting price, quantity, and expenditure.

Figure 1-4. Shifts in the Supply and Demand for Dental Care

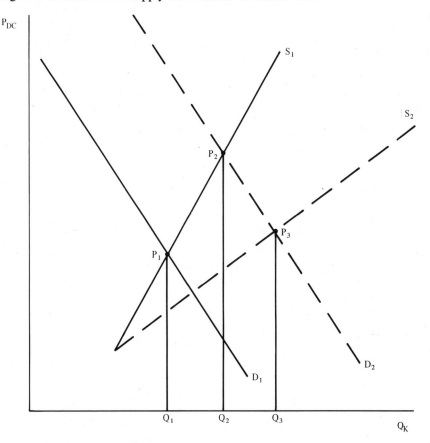

As can be seen from the two diagrams, it is important to ascertain the empirical relationships between price and quantity for both supply and demand. In other words, how much would people increase their use if price were to decline, and what would be the increase in supply if prices were to rise? Further, how much would demand (or for that matter supply) shift to the right with a change in any of the factors affecting it other than price? It is the magnitude of these relations that will determine the changes in price, quantity, and expenditure, and which is required knowledge if we are to make forecasts and to cost out different financing programs. The determination of these empirical relationships are the nature of economic research and some preliminary estimate of these will be used in this book.[1]

From the resulting demand and supply of dental care flow the demands for the inputs into the supply of dental care, the more important ones being dentists and dental auxiliaries. This suggests that in order for one to forecast demand for dental manpower one must first be able to forecast the demand for dental care, and then determine what proportion of dental care will be supplied by dentists and what proportion by auxiliaries. For example, the existing method of forecasting the number of dentists is to extrapolate the dentist-population ratio; the economic approach suggests that if demand for dental care is increased, i.e., people wish to visit the dentist more frequently, then this will increase the demand for dentists.

Maintaining the same dentist-population ratio into the future without allowing for increases in the demand for dental care will cause a rise in the price of such care and fewer visits (at a constant visit per dentist ratio) than if the ratio had been adjusted upward as a result of demand increases. Similarly, unless productivity changes in the supply of dental care are also incorporated (e.g., the greater use of dental auxiliaries), then merely extrapolating existing dentist-population ratios will result in having a larger supply of dental care than was anticipated. If federal or state dollars are to be used in financing supplies of manpower, then predictions must be more accurate to insure the better use of those funds.

The last level of the model (the first two being the market for dental care services and the market for dental inputs, primarily dentists and auxilliaries) is the demand for dentists and dental auxiliary education and the supply of that education by dental schools and auxiliary training facilities. The demand and supply of this form of education will eventually determine the quantity of inputs that comprise the supply of dental care. Hence an understanding of this market's operation and its interrelation with the rest of the system becomes crucial to the prediction of the price and quantity of dental care and the effect of policies influencing such prices and quantities.

At each level of demand and supply the determination of price and quantity occurs in what is referred to as a "market." To the extent that each of these markets is without imperfections — that consumers and providers have complete knowledge of price, quality, and productivity, and that the supply responds with increased prices for increased quantity of products or services — then the prices and quantities determined in that market will more closely approximate the true cost of producing that care and the value that consumers place on it. To the extent that there are restrictions in that market — on entry into the profession, on tasks that may be performed, on the response of the suppliers to what is demanded — then the prices and quantities determined by supply and demand will diverge from what may be considered socially optimal. Restrictions can raise prices and decrease quantities; this can and does occur in each of the markets of dental care, dental manpower, and dental education. It may be possible, therefore, to achieve the same goals that are inherent in some financing proposals by merely removing restrictions in the various dental markets.

The outcomes within each market — namely the price and quantity of dental visits in the dental care market, the wages and number of health personnel employed in the manpower market, and tuition payments and number of graduates in the education market — feed into each of the other markets and in turn affect the price and quantity in each of these other markets. It is in this way that there is a continuing relationship among levels of supply and demand in the different markets. In some markets, such as dental education, price (tuition payments) and quantity (number of graduates) may not be determined solely by the joint interaction of supply and demand. When this occurs it becomes necessary to evaluate how well this market, with its peculiar incentive systems, performs, and whether changes are indicated.

To show how the above model can be useful in a discussion on financing, let us use as an example an increase in the number of dental graduates as a result of federally funded dental school construction. The purpose of this exercise will be to predict the consequences of such a program and its cost, and then to compare these outcomes with what would result from another subsidy program, an increase in the demand for dental care as a result of a federally funded insurance program.

As an illustration of how the various levels of the dental sector are interrelated, see Figure 1-5. Charts 1, 2, and 3 show the three levels of the dental care sector under conditions of an increase in the supply of dentist training facilities. Starting with Chart 3, there is an increase in the supply of educational training facilities, e.g., more dental schools and increases in existing schools, as a result of a federal subsidy (capitation) to dental schools. If this educational market operated as would a perfectly competitive market, then the results would be similar to those shown in Chart 3A. The increase in dental school capacity, as a result of the subsidy, would be from S_1 to S_2 and would result in lower tuition rates, an increased enrollment, and hence an increased number of dental graduates. These additional graduates then represent an increase in supply (S_1 to S_2) in Chart 2. The effect of this increased supply is to reduce the wages (compared to what they would have been) from P_1 to P_2 and to have greater availability of dental manpower (Q_1 to Q_2). This increased supply of dental manpower then represents an increased input into the supply of dental care in Chart 1. The effect of the increased quantity of dental care supplied (from S_1 to S_2) in Chart 1 results in a greater quantity of dental care (Q_1 to Q_2) and lower prices (P_1 to P_2) available to the consumers.

However, the market for educational training of dentists differs from a perfectly competitive market and also from the markets for dental care and dental manpower (Charts 1 and 2). Tuition (price) and enrollments (quantity) are not determined by the interaction of the demand for and supply of dental education spaces. Instead, tuition is set by the educational institutions and quantity is limited to the available number of spaces. Thus tuition in this market is different (lower — for the same set of educational requirements) from that determined by the interaction of demand and supply. The consequence of

14

Figure 1-5. An Economic Model of the Dental Care Sector: Supply Subsidies

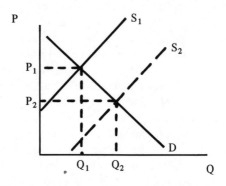

Chart 1.   Supply and Demand for Dental Care

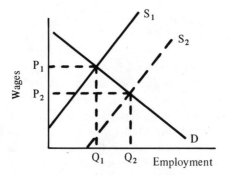

Chart 2.   Supply and Demand for Dental Manpower

(A)   (B)

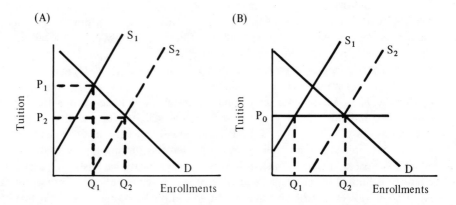

Chart 3.   Supply and Demand for Dental Training Facilities

setting tuition below the "equilibrium" level of tuition is that there is continual "excess" demand for dental school spaces.

The amount of excess demand is measured by the distance between the demand and supply curves at the fixed tuition rate. As shown in Chart 3B, at tuition rate P_0, the amount demanded will be Q_2, while the number of spaces supplied is (Q_1). The amount of excess demand is therefore $Q_2 - Q_1$, which is the number of applicants not accepted to dental schools.

In the other markets, if there were excess demand, the price would rise, there would be an increase in supply with higher prices, and an equilibrium would be established at a higher price and with an increase in quantity. However, since the dental educational market has other goals than maximizing profits or the number of students graduated, and since they are able to receive subsidies, they do not increase their tuition rates or their spaces when demand increases. Excess demand enables the schools to be more selective in their choice of applicants.[c] A subsidy to dental schools — tied to enrollment increases — would shift the supply of educational spaces from S_1 to S_2 as shown in Chart 3B. Enrollment will increase, from Q_1 to Q_2.[d]

Given the implicit objectives of dental schools, a subsidy unrelated to enrollment would probably not result in enrollment increases but rather in increased "quality" of the school. Similarly, a subsidy just to students (loans and scholarships) will not by itself increase the number of dental school spaces. A student-subsidy program will merely increase the excess demand for dental school spaces. For example, a student subsidy will lower the costs of becoming a dentist, hence shift the demand for dental education to the right as shown in Figure 1-6, Chart 3. At the same tuition rates as before the subsidy, the amount demanded would now be Q_3 and the excess demand becomes Q_3 to Q_1. The number of graduates would thus presumably not change. Thus in order to increase the supply of dental school spaces, such subsidies should be given to the school and tied to enrollment increases. Assuming the subsidy to be enrollment related, the increase in number of graduates would increase the supply in the higher levels (manpower and dental care) and the implications would be similar as described earlier.

If we wanted to describe how a change in productivity would have its effect, then we would start with Chart 1, Figure 1-5. By increased productivity we mean in an increase in the supply of dental care provided by each dentist. Hence

---

[c]The above description of the market for dental school training is different from the supply response of auxiliary training institutions. Empirical evidence on auxiliary educational institutions (presented in Chapter 4) indicates a fairly rapid response in terms of expansion of existing schools and the creation of large numbers of additional schools to increased demands for auxiliary training.

[d]The extent of the supply shift did not have to be from S_1 to S_2. For simplicity it was assumed that all subsidies to dental schools were tied to enrollment increases and that it was possible to estimate the demand at that tuition rate and desirable to eliminate any excess demand.

Figure 1-6. An Economic Model of the Dental Care Sector: Demand Subsidies

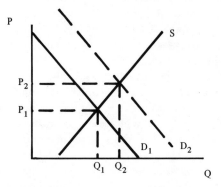

Chart 1. Supply and Demand for Dental Care

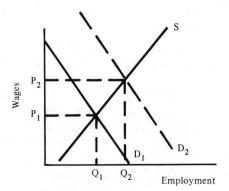

Chart 2. Supply and Demand for Dental Manpower

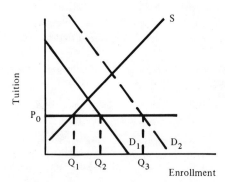

Chart 3. Supply and Demand for Dental Training Facilities

we would expect quantity to be greater — and prices lower — than if the increase in productivity had not occurred. When it is said that prices would be lower or that they would fall, this should be taken to mean lower than without such a change. It is unlikely that we would actually observe lower prices or wages since there are continuing increases in demand at each level of the sector. In order to simplify the analysis, therefore, we have held constant any increases in demand that are occurring.

Similarly, a revision of dental school curricula that would decrease the training time for dental students such that schools could graduate a greater number of dentists in a given period of time would also be represented by an increase in supply, as shown in Chart 3B. The ultimate effect of this policy in terms of price and quantity can be traced out as was done in the first example, which described the effects of an increase in the number of dental schools.

What is important here, of course, is to determine how much it costs to increase supply at any level; how much of an increase in supply is achieved; and, last, what are the ultimate effects on price and quantity in Chart 1, Figure 1-5, of an increase in supply in Chart 3. These are research questions that must be answered if we are to properly compare alternative policies, not only on the supply side but also on the demand side.

Turning to demand then, the first effect of a subsidy for the purchase of dental insurance would be to increase the demand for dental care (Figure 1-6, Chart 1). The effect of this policy (holding constant any shifts in supply elsewhere in the system) is to result in an increase in the price of care (from P_1 to P_2) and an increase in quantity (from Q_1 to Q_2). (The extent of the rise in prices and visits would depend on the elasticity of demand and supply. In order to forecast actual prices, utilization, and cost of such a program, empirical estimates of such elasticities would have to be developed.) The costs and impact of such a program would also depend upon whether it was an insurance program that subsidized part of the price of dental care or whether it just provided particular consumers with maximum dollar subsidies for dental care. If it were to pay a maximum dollar amount, then with increased prices the quantity purchased would be lower than perhaps anticipated. If it were to pay a percentage of the price of a visit, then the cost of such a program would be open-ended and would increase, since the price of a visit would have gone up.

The effect of this increased demand and higher prices shown in Chart 1 is to cause an increase in the demand for dental manpower (Chart 2). We would expect that wages and incomes of auxiliaries and dentists would also increase. Last, this initial increase in demand for dental care will eventually result in an increase in the derived demand for dental education by applicants to dental schools and to dental auxiliary training facilities, as shown in Chart 3. In the absence of additional policies to increase the supply of training facilities, the increase in demand for dental care will result in increased *excess* demand for dental school spaces. As shown in Chart 3, excess demand will increase from $Q_2 \text{-} Q_1$ to $Q_3 \text{-} Q_1$.

Both these programs — a demand subsidy to consumers or a supply subsidy to dental schools — will achieve the policy objective of increasing the quantity of dental care from Q_1 to Q_2 in Chart 1 in Figures 1-5 and 1-6. These three charts indicate the different levels at which financing programs can be undertaken. In this manner these two financing programs can be considered as alternatives and compared according to common criteria. Such diagrams may also be used to indicate the likely effects on supply and demand at each level and on prices paid by the consumer and the quantity of dental care received.

In order to compare which financing alternative is preferred, we must have additional information on who receives the additional care, how the taxes are raised to subsidize these two policies, the time it takes to achieve these changes, and the relative costs of changing demand and supply.[e] Then that subsidy program which provides the largest increase in dental care to the designated beneficiary group, for a given size of subsidy, should be preferred, other things being equal.

To summarize, the usefulness of specifying an economic model of the dental care sector is that it shows how changes in different parts of that sector are interrelated and how changes in different parts can have effects throughout the system. Such a model would suggest the data to be collected in order to conduct research on the various relationships in the model so that it can then be used for forecasting and for evaluating alternative policies through the system.

After first specifying such a model and tracing out the probable effects of different policies, an important second step is to estimate the actual magnitude of the changes that will occur throughout the system. However, in order to do this one must have data; the type to be gathered and analyzed would be suggested by the model (another reason for having a model). Then one could say what the eventual change in prices and quantities of visits would be as a result of an increase in insurance coverage or an increase in the number of dental graduates. Estimating these relationships for each part of the model is the type of research that should be undertaken if we are to forecast more accurately, to evaluate financing alternatives, and to anticipate the return to making changes in the dental care delivery system (for example, instituting measures to increase productivity). The development of an econometric model, as proposed for the dental sector, has been developed for a number of industries in our economy and, within the past few years, for the medical care sector also. The models developed for medical care, which must still be regarded as not being final because of the poor and at times unavailable data, illustrate the usefulness of such approaches for the purposes stated.[2]

Models such as the one described may be national in scope or they may be developed for use on a regional or state level. When such national models are

---

[e]For purposes of brevity and simplicity in exposition, complementary and substitution effects of changes in demand and supply have been omitted. These effects should also be considered when determining the total costs of various financing programs.

used on a state or regional level they require some modifications, primarily the inclusion of the determinants of dentists' locations.

This discussion of a model of the dental care sector should also serve as an introduction to the various markets in dental care, which will be examined in greater detail. Some empirical content will be provided to the various categories that have been up to now merely labeled "supply" and "demand."

An Overview of This Book

Up to this point, an attempt has been made to delineate the boundaries, specify objectives, and develop some criteria. The remainder of the paper is an attempt to provide a framework for further analysis, present descriptive material, and discuss some empirical work related to the objectives and criteria stated here.

Chapter 2 is an analysis of the demand for dental care. The first section analyzes the factors influencing the demand for dental care, including a discussion of dental insurance. Estimates are presented of the effect that dental prices and family incomes have on the use and expenditures for dental care. These empirical estimates are then used in later chapters on forecasting and on costing out alternative national dental insurance plans.

Chapter 3, on supply of dental services, discusses the determinants of the supply of dental services, including their distribution and use. Data on the stock of dentists are presented, together with a discussion of their accuracy. The various indices used to measure dental productivity and estimates of the change in each of these measures over time are presented with estimates of the percent of capacity at which the dental services industry has been operating. Estimates of the rate of return to a dental education as one determinant of the long run supply of dental services are developed, as well as the sensitivity of the rate of return to changes in its various conponents.

Chapter 4 is an analysis of the market for dental and auxiliary education. The responsiveness of these educational institutions to increased demands for training are examined as well as the possible existence of economies of scale in dental schools. A preliminary evaluation is made of the Health Professions Education Act in order to determine who are the main beneficiaries of this legislation, what has been its impact, and how accurate were the bases upon which it was started.

Chapter 5 describes the development and application of an econometric model of the dental sector for use in forecasting and policy evaluation. A simulation analysis was conducted in order to forecast the effects of future changes in demand on dental prices, visits, expenditures, and dental incomes. Using the econometric model, the policy implications of maintaining a constant dentist-to-population ratio are evaluated, as well as various proposals to increase the supply of dental care, such as the Health Professions Education Act to subsidize an increase in the number of dentists.

Chapter 6 is a discussion of the government role in the dental sector. Economic criteria are presented for the different roles of government and the method of financing called for under each. Included in this chapter is a discussion of differing values in income redistribution and the reasons for government intervention on grounds of economic efficiency. The results of a simulation program that attempted to estimate the expenditures and visits under alternative national insurance plans for dental care are also given.

Chapter 7 contains a summary and some concluding observations.

2

The Demand for Personal
Dental Care

Personal Expenditures on Dental Care

Dental care is primarily a personal decision. An individual or family decides on
how much and what kind of dental care services they are willing to buy. In order
to forecast personal dental care expenditures and utilization, therefore, it is
necessary to understand and predict the magnitudes of those factors affecting
the demand and supply of dental care. The consequences of financing of such
care can then be predicted and its effects on utilization, expenditure, and price
can be forecast within such a supply and demand framework.

However, all dental care is not personal in the sense of individuals or
households making the decisions. The fluoridation of water supplies in a
community or expenditures on research to eliminate oral disease are "public"
decisions; they are beyond the control of any one household and are more in the
nature of community or aggregate level decisions. The level and composition of
the financing of "public" programs is also important and should be analyzed
separately from discussions of financing personal dental care. The criterion for
separating such decisions is based on who potentially benefits from the program.
In the "public" case all individuals, whether or not they were in favor of such a
program, receive the potential benefits from it, since public goods are indivisible;
one person's consumption does not prevent other persons from potentially
benefiting from it, therefore they should all participate in the financing.

Personal dental care, on the other hand, primarily benefits those who receive
it, therefore the financing decision is undertaken primarily by those who benefit.
If a program supplements the demand and use of personal dental care then this is
basically an income redistribution program. That is, a value judgment is made to
devote more resources to meeting the dental needs of various population groups
in society (classified by criteria such as age or income). The criteria involved in
financing such income redistribution programs should be based upon ability to
pay. Generally the recipients of such programs should receive care the value of
which is greater than their contribution to the taxes required to pay for it
(which may be zero), while those subsidizing it should pay taxes that are more
than the value of such additional care they receive from such a program (which
may be zero). Further, the persons subsidizing such programs should have higher
incomes than the recipients.

In order, therefore, to evaluate these basically different types of financing
programs (personal versus "public") and to make forecasts of expenditures
under each, they should be separately analyzed. This discussion should not be

21

interpreted as meaning that even though the financing analyses should be separated, that what is done in the "public" dental sector is separate from the personal dental care sector; they are, in fact, interrelated. For example, increased expenditures on fluoridated water supplies will increase the demand for some form of personal dental care. Presumably, research on oral disease will also affect the level and composition of the demand for dental care.

Unfortunately, data on dental expenditures are not presented in this manner. Table 2-1 shows total expenditures on dental care from 1940 to 1970. The public and private categorization used in this table is different from the private and public distinction just made. In this table personal expenditures are not separated from those that are public in nature, i.e., that potentially benefit more than the user of personal dental services; rather, they are separated on the basis

Table 2-1. Private and Governmental Expenditures for Dental Care, 1940-1970 (In Thousands)

Year	Per Cent of Disposable Personal Income[1]	Total Expenditures	Consumers	Federal	State & Local
1970[2]	0.65%	$4,440,000	$4,211,000	$133,000	$ 96,000
1969[2]	0.64	4,047,000	3,830,000	120,000	98,000
1968[2]	0.61	3,623,000	3,379,000	127,000	117,000
1967[3]	0.62	3,360,000	3,235,000	70,000	56,000
1966[3]	0.58	2,964,000	2,907,000	28,000	28,000
1965[4]	0.59	2,808,000	2,773,000	16,000	19,000
1964[4]	0.60	2,648,000	2,615,000	14,000	18,000
1963[4]	0.56	2,277,000	2,250,000	13,000	14,000
1962[4]	0.58	2,234,000	2,210,000	13,000	12,000
1961[5]	0.57	2,068,000	2,048,000	10,000	10,000
1960[5]	0.56	1,977,000	1,962,000	7,000	8,000
1955[5]	0.55	1,525,000	1,508,000	13,000	4,000
1950[5]	0.47	975,000	961,000	11,000	3,000
1940[6]	0.55	419,000	419,000	---	---

Sources:

1. *Statistical Abstract of the United States,* various editions (income data).

2. Cooper, Barbara S., and Worthington, Nancy L., *National Health Expenditures, Calendar Years 1929-70,* Social Security Administration, Office of Research and Statistics, Research and Statistics Note No. 1, January 14, 1972.

3. Cooper, Barbara S., *National Health Expenditures, Fiscal Years 1929-69 and Calendar Years 1929-1968,* Social Security Administration, Office of Research and Statistics, Note No. 18, November 7, 1969.

4. Rice, Dorothy, and Cooper, Barbara S., "National Health Expenditures 1950-66," *Social Security Bulletin,* April, 1968.

5. Hanft, Ruth S., "National Health Expenditures, 1950-65," *Social Security Bulletin,* February, 1967.

6. Cooper, Barbara S., *National Health Expenditures, 1929-67,* Social Security Administration, Office of Research and Statistics, Research and Statistics Note No. 16, September 29, 1969.

of who pays for the care. On this basis it is predominantly a private sector with the contribution from governmental sources being approximately 5 percent of the total (which includes both "public" care and public financing of private care).

Expenditures on dental care, from both private and governmental sources, have been increasing over time. As a percent of disposable personal income, dental expenditures are less than 1 percent (acutally .065) − a small portion of the consumer's budget. This percentage is, however, increasing. Expenditures from governmental sources, still representing a small percentage of total dental expenditures, have increased in the last several years, primarily from the introduction of Medicaid.

Yearly data on national dental expenditures are estimated and compiled by the Social Security Administration. The basis for these estimates are data supplied by the Internal Revenue Service based on the income tax returns of dentists. (A more complete discussion of this data is provided in the notes to Table 2-2.) Estimates of dental expenditures from these sources place total consumer expenditure on dental care at approximately $4.2 billion in 1970. There have, however, been several national surveys at different periods of time which have collected data on dental expenditures; estimates from these surveys suggest that the published data on dental expenditures by SSA are understated by as much as 20 to 50 percent.

The National Center for Health Statistics, Department of Health, Education, and Welfare, as part of their Health Interview Survey, collected data on consumer expenditure for dental care in 1962. These estimates are approximately $1.3 billion (or 60 percent) higher than those published by SSA for that year. The National Opinion Research Center, University of Chicago, conducted a survey of dental care in the United States for 1964. Their estimates also exceeded those of SSA by approximately $800 million (or 30 percent). Three additional nationwide surveys of medical care utilization were conducted by the National Opinion Research Center in 1953, 1958, and 1963. Consumer expenditure on dental care, as estimated by these surveys, also consistently exceeded the published estimates by SSA for those same time periods. The American Dental Association in its periodic *Surveys of Dental Practice,* which collect data from the dentist rather than the consumer as in the above nationwide surveys, also provided estimates that exceeded those of the Social Security Administration. The data from these different sources are summarized in Table 2-2. It is extremely difficult to gather accurate data on consumer expenditures for many services, particularly ones that represent a small portion of the consumer's budget. However, uncertainties as to the true magnitude of such expenditures make it difficult to develop accurate forecasts as well as to estimate the possible substitution of government for private sources as new dental programs are introduced.

Dental expenditures will increase if for no other reason than because of increases in the population. Therefore, when examined on a per capita basis we

Table 2-2. Comparison of "Consumer Expenditures for Dental Care" from Various Sources (In Thousands)

Year	H.E.W.[1]	S.S.A.[2]	N.O.R.C.[3]	H.I.F.[4]	A.D.A.[5]
1970		$4,211,000			$6,146,070
1969		3,830,000			
1968		3,379,000			
1967		3,235,000			4,577,399
1966		2,907,000			
1965		2,773,000			
1964		2,615,000	$3,439,530		3,366,086
1963		2,250,000		$2,700,000	
1962	$3,529,022	2,210,000			
1961		2,048,000			2,650,916
1960		1,962,000			
1958				2,400,000	2,262,865
1955		1,508,000			1,844,964
1953				1,600,000	1,506,447
1950		961,000			

Notes:

1. *Source:* U.S. Department of Health, Education and Welfare, Public Health Service, *Medical Care, Health Status and Family Income, United States,* PHS Publication No. 1000 – Series 10, No. 9, Washington, D.C., 1964, p. 48. Data collected by personal interview survey. Total expenditures calculated by multiplying per-capita expenditure by "Total Resident Population" as stated in *Statistical Abstract of the United States.*

2. *Sources:* 1950-1961: Hanft, Ruth S., "National Health Expenditures 1950-1965," *Social Security Bulletin,* February 1967; 1962-1965: Rice, Dorothy, and Barbara S. Cooper, "National Health Expenditures 1950-66," *Social Security Bulletin,* April 1968; 1966-1967: Cooper, Barbara S., *National Health Expenditures, Fiscal Years 1929-1969 and Calendar Years 1929-1968,* Social Security Administration, Office of Research and Statistics, Note No. 18, November 7, 1969; 1968-1970: Cooper, Barbara S., and Nancy L. Worthington, *National Health Expenditures, Calendar Years 1929-1970,* Social Security Administration, Office of Research and Statistics, Research and Statistics Note No. 1, January 14, 1972.

Figures are compiled as follows: The estimates of expenditures for the services of dentists in private practice are based on the gross incomes from self-employment practices reported by dentists on Schedule C of the income tax return. The data include gross incomes of sole proprietorships, partnerships, offices organized as corporations, dental laboratories (estimated), and the estimated expenses of group practice prepayment plans in providing dentists' services. The salaries of dentists on hospital and hospital outpatient staffs, in Indian Health, activities in field services of the Armed Forces, and expenditures for education and training of personnel, are *not* included. The gross receipts of dentists thus represent total expenditures for these services. Consumer payments are estimated as a residual by deducting vendor payments under government programs and estimated payments to physicians and dentists from philanthropic agencies. There is a lag of one year between the current year figure and the I.R.S. data used; an upward revision is made based upon current year fee data and past relationships between fees and dentist incomes. The estimated figures are later corrected when actual data for the year becomes available.

The Social Security Administration estimates that in recent years, these figures have been increasingly understated due to failure to include incomes of corporate dental practitioners (recent legislation has made it more advantageous to the dentist to incorporate himself). It is estimaed that in 1970 this results in a downward bias of about $500,000,000.

3. *Source:* Anderson, O.W., and Newman, John F., *Patterns of Dental Service Utilization in the United States: A Nationwide Social Survey,* University of Chicago Center for Health

Administration Studies, Research Series #30, 1972. Data collected by personal interview survey. Total expenditures calculated by multiplying per-capita expenditure by "Total Resident Population" as stated in *Statistical Abstract of the United States.*

4. *Sources:* 1952-1953, 1957-1958: Anderson, O.W., Collette, Patricia, and Feldman, J. J., *Changes in Family Medical Care Expenditures and Voluntary Health Insurance.* Harvard University Press, Cambridge, 1963. 1963: Andersen, Ronald, and Anderson, O.W., *A Decade of Health Services,* University of Chicago Press, Chicago, 1967. Data collected by personal interview survey.

5. *Figure:* Calculated by multiplying "mean gross income of independent dentists" by "active practicing dentists". Source for income data: ADA., *Survey of Dental Practice,* 1953, 1956, 1959, 1962, 1965, 1968, 1971. Source for dentist supply data: U.S. Department of Health, Education and Welfare, Public Health Service, Division of Dental Health, *Health Manpower Source Book: Section 20, Manpower Supply and Educational Statistics,* updated to March, 1971. P.H.S. Publication No. 263, Section 20. Some of the "active dentist" figures used are interpolations on available actual data. The ADA data is biased upward relative to the S.S.A. – data in that the former reflects income received by dentists from government agencies (e.g., Medicaid) whereas the latter does not.

observe that consumer expenditures on dental care have still been increasing over time. On a per capita basis, therefore, expenditures can increase because of increases in either prices, quantity, or both. One reason for the rise in dental expenditures has been the increased price of dental care. For example, since 1950 the price of dental care has risen more rapidly than the Consumer Price Index (CPI) (see Table 2-3). From 1950 to 1960 the increase in dental fees has been approximately the same as the CPI (and slightly less than the rise in physician fees). From 1960 to 1970, however, while the CPI has risen from 88.7 to 116.3, dental fees have increased from 81.9 to 120.3. (During that same period, physician fees increased from 77.0 to 121.4.) When per capita dental expenditures are adjusted for increases in the price of dental care, as shown in Table 2-4, per capita expenditures have still increased, although at a much slower rate.

The increase in adjusted per capita dental expenditures has been 2.2 percent per year from 1955 to 1970 (or a total of 38 percent), while the increase in unadjusted per capita expenditures has been 5.6 percent per year, or a total of 126 percent.

Another way of looking at the increase in per capita purchases of dental care is to examine the increase in visits per capita over time. As shown in Table 2-5, estimates of dental visits are available from several sources, primarily from the National Center for Health Statistics and the American Dental Association. Although there are differences between these sources, they are slight, except for the more recent years where the ADA data are approximately 20 percent greater than that of the National Center for Health Statistics. The increase in visits per capita (ADA data) has been 1.2 percent from 1955 to 1970, or a total of 20 percent.

The rise in adjusted (for price changes) per capita dental expenditures may have been a result of a number of factors, such as a change in the age distribution of the population, changes in per capita income, or even a change in the composition of a dental visit. Offsetting such increases in per capita

26

Table 2-3. Consumer, Medical, Physician, and Dental Price Indices — 1935-1971 (1967 = 100)[1]

Year	CPI	Medical Care Price Index	M.D. Fees	Dental Care Price Index			
				Dentist Fees	Fillings, Adult, 1 Surface	Extractions, Adult	Complete Upper Denture
1971	121.3	128.4	129.8	127.0	128.0	126.9	124.9
1970	116.3	120.6	121.4	119.4	120.3	118.6	118.3
1969	109.8	113.4	112.9	112.9	113.1	112.9	112.3
1968	104.2	106.1	105.6	105.5	105.4	105.2	106.1
1967	100.0	100.0	100.0	100.0	100.0	100.0	100.0
1966	97.2	93.4	93.4	95.2	94.7	96.7	94.9
1965	94.5	89.5	88.3	92.2	91.3	93.9	92.2
1964	92.9	87.3	85.2	89.4	88.8	90.4	89.7
1963	91.7	85.6	83.1	87.1	86.8	87.4	—[2]
1962	90.6	83.5	81.3	84.7	84.3	85.0	—
1961	89.6	81.4	79.0	82.5	82.0	83.1	—
1960	88.7	79.1	77.0	82.1	81.9	82.0	—
1955	80.2	64.8	65.4	73.0	72.5	73.8	—
1950	72.1	53.7	55.2	63.9	63.9	62.8	—
1940	42.0	36.8	39.6	42.0	42.1	40.3	—
1935	41.1	36.1	39.2	40.8	40.4	39.5	—

1. *Source:* Martin Smith, U.S. Department of Labor, Bureau of Labor Statistics.
2. "Complete Upper Denture" not compiled before 1964.

expenditures has been the rise in dental prices over time, which has undoubtedly reduced per capita purchases of dental care.

In order to understand and be able to forecast expenditures in the aggregate as well as on a per capita basis, therefore, it becomes important to understand and forecast the determinants of dental price and quantity. In this way we can suggest what is likely to happen to demand for dental care and, subsequently, to the supply of dental care. It should then be possible to combine both of these analyses to make some forecasts of price, quantity, and expenditure under different financing programs.

The Demand for Dental Care

There have been many studies on the determinants of utilization of dental services.[1] These studies have employed various methodologies in the analysis of primarily survey data; and both economic as well as noneconomic variables have been used to explain observed differentials in use of dental care. No attempt will be made here to provide a complete review of the literature in this area; instead, an economic approach to the study of demand will be presented, together with the type of information that an economist requires if he is to be able to predict and explain differences in demand, (the purposes of demand analysis). It should be remembered that actual use of services depends upon both demand *and* supply. Just having an estimate of demand will not enable us to predict use unless we also have some estimates of the likely supply of those services.

Table 2-4. Per Capita Consumer Expenditures for Dental Care

Year	Per Capita Dental Expenditures	Adjusted Per Capita Dental Expenditures
1970	$20.67	$17.31
1969	18.94	16.78
1968	16.98	16.09
1967	16.39	16.39
1966	15.14	15.90
1965	14.33	15.54
1964	13.69	15.31
1963	11.94	13.71
1962	11.90	14.05
1961	11.27	13.66
1960	10.97	13.36
1955	9.14	12.52
1950	6.33	9.91
1940	3.16	7.52

Source: Table 2.1 and Table 2.3.

Table 2-5. Dental Visits, Total and Per Capita: A Comparison of Three Sources

Year	HEW[1]		ADA[2]		NORC[3]	
	Total	Per Capita	Total	Per Capita	Total	Per Capita
1970	303,552,000	1.5	369,334,000	1.81		
1969	293,337,000	1.5				
1968	259,990,000	1.3				
1967			358,073,430	1.81		
1964			309,551,771	1.62	286,627,500	1.5
1963	293,750,000	1.6				
1961			280,897,140	1.54		
1958	258,000,000	1.6	272,100,290	1.56		
1955			248,606,293	1.51		
1952			230,170,696	1.47		

1. *Sources:* 1958: U.S. Department of Health, Education, and Welfare, Public Health Service, *Health Statistics From the U.S. National Health Survey: Dental Care, Volume of Visits, United States, July 1957 – June 1959,* Series B, No. 15, Washington D.C. April 1960, p. 17; 1963: U.S. Department of Health, Education, and Welfare, *Volume of Dental Visits, United States, July 1963 – June 1964.* Public Health Service Publication No. 1000–Series 10, No. 23, Washington, D.C., October 1965, p. 18; 1968-1970: U.S. Department of Health, Education, and Welfare, Public Health Service, *Current Estimates from the Health Interview Survey, United States, 1968, 1969, 1970.* PHS Publication No. 1000–Series 10, Nos. 60, 63, 72. Data collected by personal interview.

2. Calculated by multiplying "mean patient visits per dentist" by "active practicing dentists." Source for mean visit data: ADA, *Survey of Dental Practice,* 1953, 1956, 1959, 1962, 1965, 1968, 1971. Source for dentist supply data: U.S. Department of Health, Education, and Welfare, Public Health Service, Division of Dental Health, *Health Manpower Source Book: Section 20, Manpower Supply and Educational Statistics,* updated to March 1971. PHS Publication No. 263, Section 20. Some of the "active dentist" figures used are interpolations on available actual data.

3. *Source:* Anderson, O.W., and Newman, John F., *Patterns of Dental Service Utilization in the United States: A Nationwide Social Survey,* University of Chicago Center for Health Administration Studies, Research Series #30, 1972. Data collected by personal interview survey. Total visits calculated by multiplying per capita visits by "Total Resident Population," as given in *Statistical Abstract of the United States.*

The Determinants of Demand

Analyses of the demand for dental care attempt to estimate the determinants of dental care use at different prices. The price of dental care is therefore one determinant of demand and forecasts of future demand must be made with some estimate in mind of the price of care. If all of the other determinants of demand were unchanged, but the price were to vary, then the demand for dental care would also vary.

The major categories of factors other than price that are believed to influence demand for dental care are the need for such care in the population, attitudes toward dental care and oral hygiene practices, and economic factors (income, the prices of related medical services, public funds spent for the purchase of dental services, the existence of dental insurance). Thus one could visualize a "demand function" that related the quantity of dental care demanded to these determinants.

An analysis of demand must not only ascertain whether a factor is a determinant of demand, but also what effect that factor has on influencing demand. Although a number of important factors affect the demand for dental care other than just the price of that care, it is still important to determine the effect of price if we are to predict future demand or if we want to change a person's demand for care. The responsiveness of changes in demand to changes in price is called "price elasticity of demand." The impact of deductibles and copayments under insured dental care, for example, is related to the price elasticity of demand. This will be discussed more fully below.

It is necessary to realize that even if the price of dental care were zero for all persons or just for low income groups, the utilization of dental care by low income families would not be the same as that of high income groups. There are several reasons for this; attitudes toward seeking dental care would probably still differ between income groups, and there would still be additional costs associated with dental use that do not disappear even though the price of that care is zero. Examples of such costs are travel and waiting time and travel cost to the dentist's office, which are probably greater for low income persons. Dentists are probably located in closer proximity to higher income areas and although this might change as demand for care is increased in low income areas, until then low income persons might still incur travel costs that would be a deterrent, as was price, to seeking care. Similarly, low income persons are less apt to be reimbursed for time lost from work when visiting a dentist than are higher income persons. Because of the existence of these travel costs and time lost from work, the poor are likely to have a lower "price elasticity of demand" than higher income persons; lowering the price of dental care to the poor is not likely to achieve as large an increase in demand as it would for the more affluent.

An economist is not just interested in measuring the effect of different prices on utilization of services, nor in only economic factors, because unless the major determinants are identified and estimated it will not be possible to provide accurate forecasts of future use. It is important to ascertain the net effect of each of the major factors affecting demand (by forecasting how each one of these factors will change) if we are to estimate future demand. If it is desired to change a person's demand for care, we must know the effect of changing any of the factors affecting demand. Demands for dental care can be changed by changing any number of factors; however, it will cost different amounts to change each factor (e.g., increasing consumer's dental knowledge versus lowering the price of dental care), and the change in demand will differ depending upon which factor is changed. For a given budget, therefore, to achieve a change in demand at lowest cost it is important to know the cost of changing each demand determinant as well as its effect on quantity demanded. Demand studies — generally through the use of some form of multivariate analysis — attempt to provide part of this information, namely, the effect on demand of each of the major determinants, whether they are economic or noneconomic variables.

Each of these major determinants of demand will be briefly discussed.

The Need for Dental Care

Other things being equal, it is presumed that persons with greater need for dental care would have greater use and expenditures for dental care than persons with fewer needs. According to one nationwide survey of dental use, when dental symptoms are present, expenditures and visits are approximately twice as great within each age, sex, or racial category. Data showing the percent of persons with various dental symptoms and the proportion of those persons seeing a dentist are presented in Table 2-6. The presence or absence of dental symptoms,

Table 2-6. Distribution of Dental Conditions and the Proportion of Persons with Conditions Who Made a Dental Visit

Condition	Proportion with Condition	Proportion with Condition Who Made a Visit
Toothache	20% (9330)	75% (1401)
Sore or bleeding gums	8% (9302)	45% (698)
Loose permanent tooth	5% (9321)	61% (451)
Pain in tooth when drinking hot or cold liquid	14% (9302)	54% (1256)
Tartar or stains on teeth	25% (9255)	57% (2363)
Crooked teeth	7% (9311)	32% (698)

Source: Newman, John F., and Anderson, O.W., *Patterns of Dental Service Utilization in the United States: A Nationwide Social Survey,* Center for Health Administration Studies, The University of Chicago, 1972, p. 84.

however, does not account for all the variation in dental use or expenditure. When the effect of other factors to be discussed, such as income or education, are considered, we then observe a stronger relationship between the presence of symptoms and a dental visit.

Data on dental symptoms are generally not available and other measures are used to indicate the relative need for dental care in the population. An example of such a variable is the age distribution of the population in a community. As age increases, the number of visits per person increases until 15 to 24 years of age and then slowly declines with increased age. This inverted "U" shape between visits and age can be seen from the data presented in Table 2-7. The age-visit relationship appears to be fairly consistent for the four different time periods for which data are available. The type of dental treatment which will be demanded also varies according to age. As shown in Table 2-8, there is proportionately greater demand for fillings, cleanings, examinations, and straightening among the younger ages, while the older age groups have greater demands for denture work and gum treatment. Thus, when age is related to expenditures on dental care, the relationship is consistently positive, rather than being similar to the age-visit relationship. Although the visit rate for older age groups is lower, the type of treatment being demanded is more expensive. Therefore, expenditures on dental care increase with age.

Additional variables representing differential needs for dental care would be sex, urban-rural, white/nonwhite, and whether or not the water supply in the community is fluoridated. With regard to this latter variable, it is expected that fluoridation would result primarily in a decrease in the need for treatment of caries among children, hence a lower demand for this particular type of dental care.

There has been a great deal of evidence on the effect of fluoridation on tooth decay in children. A summary of some of these studies suggests that fluoridated water supplies will prevent up to two-thirds of the tooth decay in children. The cost of providing dental care to children in nonfluoridated areas is more than twice as high as for children in fluoridated areas: Estimates of the cost of providing dental care for children in tax-supported programs such as Head Start show per child costs from two to four times higher per child than in fluoridated areas.[2]

In addition to decreasing the need, hence demand for dental care, communities with fluoridated water supplies would have a different composition of "needs" for dental care than would nonfluoridated areas. A recently published study comparing dental practices in fluoridated and fluoride deficient areas show that dentists working in fluoridated areas serve a larger patient load (lower dentist-population ratio), felt less overworked, spent more time on each patient sitting, and earned larger incomes. Differences in the nature of the treatments provided are slight, but dentists in fluoridated areas provided more restorations to their younger patients, while in the fluoride deficient areas there was a greater likelihood of extractions in the same age group. Specialty treatment also constituted a larger proportion of treatments in the fluoridated communities.[3]

The cost savings of having fluoridated water supplies have been demonstrated almost as frequently as has the decrease in caries. It has been estimated that the cost of fluoridation is approximately 10 cents per year per person.[4] On purely economic grounds, therefore, there would be large cost savings both to families and to governmental programs providing dental care to children if the community's water supplies were fluoridated.[5]

Table 2-7. Number of Dental Visits per Person per Year by Age

Both Sexes	1957-1958[1]		1963-1964[2]		1968[3]		1969[4]	
	Total	Per Capita	Total	Per Capita	Total	Per Capita	Total	Per Capita
All Ages	258,500,000	1.5	293,750,000	2.1	259,990,000	1.4	293,337,000	1.5
Under 5 Yrs.	5,200,000	0.3	6,893,000	0.3	5,623,000	0.6	5,267,000	0.3
5-14	61,700,000	1.8	71,642,000	1.9	65,061,000	1.6	74,759,000	1.8
15-24	47,400,000	2.2	53,844,000	2.0	54,618,000	1.7	56,340,000	1.7
25-44	80,200,000	1.8	84,498,000	1.9	63,436,000	1.4	74,053,000	1.6
45-64	52,300,000	1.5	63,228,000	1.7	54,290,000	1.3	63,899,000	1.6
65 & over	11,600,000	0.8	13,644,000	0.8	16,962,000	0.9	19,018,000	1.0

1. *Source:* Department of Health, Education, and Welfare, *Health Statistics from the U.S. National Health Survey: Dental Care, Volume of Visits, United States, July 1957 – June 1959,* Series B-No. 15, Washington, D.C., April 1960, pp. 12-13.

2. *Source:* Department of Health, Education, and Welfare, *Volume of Dental Visits, United States, July 1963 – June 1964* Public Health Service Publication No. 1000—Series 10, No. 23, Washington, D.C., October 1965, p. 17.

3. *Source:* Department of Health, Education, and Welfare, Public Health Service, *Monthly Vital Statistics Report: Health – Interview Survey – Provisional Data from the National Center for Health Statistics,* Vol. 18, No. 9, Supplement 2, December 18, 1969, pp. 4-5.

4. *Source:* Unpublished Data from the *Health Interview Survey,* National Center for Health Statistics, Public Health Service, Department of Health, Education, and Welfare, Rockville, Maryland.

Table 2-8. Percent Distribution of Dental Visits by Type of Service According to Age

Type of Service	All Ages		0 – 4		5 – 14		15 – 24		25 – 44		45 – 64		65+	
	1957-58[1]	1963-64[4]	1957-58[1]	1963-64[4]	1957-58[1]	1963-64[4]	1957-58[1]	1963-64[4]	1957-58[1]	1963-64[4]	1957-58[1]	1963-64[4]	1957-58[1]	1963-64[4]
Fillings	43.0	37.8	43.7	37.0	49.9	41.3	54.5	45.0	42.3	39.1	32.3	29.9	16.7	20.3
Extractions	17.0	15.0	8.2	4.5	12.2	11.7	18.5	15.6	19.4	16.5	17.3	16.8	21.9	17.0
Cleaning/Examination	17.7	34.7	30.6	63.1	18.1	38.9	11.9	30.6	19.4	35.3	18.4	31.5	15.7	24.9
Straightening	3.4	5.8	–[2]	–[3]	9.2	15.9	4.7	9.3	1.2	–[3]	0.3	–[3]	–[2]	–[3]
Gum Treatment	1.5	3.6	–[2]	–[3]	0.6	1.1	0.9	3.0	2.5	5.3	1.9	4.8	1.1	3.7
Denture Work	8.6	13.2	1.1	–[3]	1.4	1.5	3.7	5.5	6.7	15.0	19.0	25.7	34.5	41.5
Other/Unknown	12.3	–	22.2	–	12.6	–	8.4	–	13.1	–	13.1	–	12.1	–
Total[5]	100.0	100.0	100.0	100.0	100.0	100.0	100.0	100.0	100.0	100.0	100.0	100.0	100.0	100.0

1. *Source*: Department of Health, Education, and Welfare, *Health Statistics from the U.S. National Health Survey; Dental Care, Volume of Visits, United States, July 1957 – June 1959.* Series B-No. 15, Washington, D.C., April 1969, p. 26.

2. Quantity is zero.

3. Figure does not meet standards of reliability or precision.

4. *Source*: Department of Health, Education, and Welfare, *Volume of Dental Visits, United States, July 1963 – June 1964,* Public Health Service Publication No. 1000—Series 10, No. 23, Washington, D.C., October 1965, p. 34.

5. Figures may add to more than 100% because more than one type of service may be performed during a single visit.

As of 1969, according to *Fluoridation Census* (National Institute of Health, U.S. Department of Health, Education, and Welfare), approximately 43 percent of the population was using fluoridated water supplies; this is an increase from 29 percent in 1964. In terms of the percent of central water systems that use fluoridated waters, less than 30 percent do so. The communities that are more likely to have fluoridated water supplies are the larger metropolitan areas, while it is the small rural communities that are more likely to be fluoride deficient. The percent of all communities of different sizes having fluoridated water is shown in Table 2-9.

It would appear therefore that there are still high returns to be expected from having fluoridated water supplies extended to those communities served by a central water supply that are currently without fluoridation. (The reasons for communities not having fluoridation are varied, but cost of doing so would certainly be one factor.)

To summarize the discussion on need for dental care, persons having dental symptoms, and hence greater needs for care, are more likely, other things being equal, to see a dentist than those who do not have such symptoms. Need as one factor affecting demand for care is also more likely among the younger age groups. The extension of preventive measures, such as fluoridation and good oral hygiene habits, would serve to decrease the need for care, and hence be one factor decreasing the demand for care. It is likely that these preventive measures will continue to increase in the future and should therefore serve to decrease the demand for dental care primarily among the younger age groups.

Attitudes Toward Dental Care and Oral Hygiene Practices

If need for dental care and economic status were similar for different persons but the people differed in their attitudes and knowledge regarding dental care, we would then expect to observe different use rates among them. A measure that has often been used to represent differing attitudes toward seeking dental care and practicing proper dental hygiene are the number of years of education of the head of the household. Years of formal education is not an entirely satisfactory measure; it is strongly related to other factors such as family income, white/nonwhite, and urbanization. It thus becomes difficult to measure the net effect that purely attitudinal factors and knowledge have on the demand for dental care without including the effect of economic factors at the same time.

Table 2-10 shows the number of visits per person when the data are classified by both family income and education of the head of the household. Within each income classification there is a higher utilization rate for those persons where the head of household has more years of education. As can be seen from the table, however, the major differences in utilization rates are between income groupings, rather than between levels of education.

Table 2-9. Percent of All Communities Using Controlled Fluoridation, by Size of Community[1]

Size of Community[2]	Total Communities	Dec. 31, 1964		Dec. 31, 1965		Dec. 31, 1967		Dec. 31, 1969	
		Number Using	Percent	Number Using	Percent	Number Using	Percent	Number Using	Percent
All	20,582	2758	13.4	3030	14.7	3827	18.6	4834	23.5
1,000,000 and over	5	2	40.0	3	60.0	4	80.0	4	80.0
500,000 – 999,999	16	8	50.0	8	50.0	9	56.2	11	68.8
250,000 – 499,999	30	13	43.3	13	43.3	14	46.7	16	53.3
100,000 – 249,999	81	30	37.0	33	40.7	43	53.1	47	58.0
50,000 – 99,999	201	75	37.3	81	40.2	103	51.2	109	54.2
25,000 – 49,999	433	148	34.2	164	38.0	222	51.4	250	57.9
10,000 – 24,999	1133	400	35.3	454	40.0	570	50.3	637	56.2
5,000 – 9,999	1398	439	31.4	489	35.1	588	42.2	665	47.7
2,500 – 4,999	2145	429	20.0	487	22.6	563	26.2	709	32.9
1,000 – 2,499	4452	512	11.5	585	13.1	732	16.4	931	20.8
Under 1,000 and not specified	10,636	702	6.6	713	6.7	979	9.2	1455	13.6

1. *Source:* U.S. Department of Health, Education, and Welfare, Public Health Service, National Institute of Health, *Fluoridation Census,* 1965, 1966, 1968, 1969. U.S. Government Printing Office, Washington, D.C.

2. Populations based on 1960 census.

Table 2-10. Number of Dental Visits, and Dental Visits per Capita, by Family Income and Education of Head of Family

1963-1964 Education

Income	Under 9 Years		9-12 Years		13+ Years	
	Total(000)	Per Capita	Total(000)	Per Capita	Total(000)	Per Capita
Under $4,000	18,005	0.7	16,822	0.9	7,027	1.8
$4,000 – $6,900	18,753	1.1	48,398	1.5	17,430	2.0
$7,000 – $9,999	9,486	1.4	37,378	1.9	22,991	2.4
$10,000 and above	6,931	2.0	27,348	2.3	46,674	3.5
All Incomes	56,690	1.0	136,911	1.6	97,242	2.6

1969 Education

Income	Under 5 Years		5-8 Years		9-11 Years		12 Years		13+ Years	
	Total(000)	Per Capita	Total(000)	Per Capita	Total(000)	Per Capita	Total(000)	Per Capita	Total(000)	P.C.
Under $5,000	3,481	0.6	10,389	0.7	8,309	0.9	10,097	1.2	7,597	1.7
$5,000 and above	2,393	0.7	22,257	1.0	35,565	1.4	80,651	1.6	93,414	2.3
All Incomes	6,342	0.6	35,688	0.9	46,416	1.3	95,749	1.6	106,048	2.2

Source: Unpublished data from the Health Interview Survey, National Center for Health Statistics, Department of Health, Education, and Welfare.

Economic Factors Affecting the Demand for Dental Care

Even though there may be a need and a desire for dental care, there may be little or no actual use because of inadequate ability to purchase such care. One of these economic factors, the price of dental care, was discussed earlier. The other economic variables which should be included in any demand analysis are family income, the prices of related medical services, the amount of public funds spent for the purchase of dental services, and the availability of dental insurance. Persons with larger incomes are able to purchase more of all goods and services including more dental care and care of a higher quality.

Based upon cross tabulations of survey data, as shown in Table 2-11, persons with higher incomes have much higher utilization rates than do those with lower incomes. (Higher income families are also more likely to purchase dental insurance, as will be discussed below.) The type of dental treatment demanded will also vary according to family income. According to Table 2-12, lower income families will have a greater proportionate demand for dentures and extractions than will higher income families. Those with higher incomes are likely to demand proportionately more preventive and maintenance work, i.e., fillings, examinations, cleanings, straightenings, and gum treatment.

The availability of public programs to finance the purchase or provision of dental care (directly or indirectly) will also serve to increase the overall demand for such care, although the proportion of demand that is privately versus governmentally financed may shift.

Table 2-11. Dental Visits per Person per Year by Family Income

Family Income	1957-1959[1]	1963-1964[2]	1968[3]	1969[4]
$ 0 – $ 1999	.7	.8	–	–
$ 0 – $ 2999	–	–	.9	.8
$ 2000 – $ 3999	1.0	.9	–	–
$ 3000 – $ 4999	–	–	.9	1.0
$ 4000 – $ 6999	1.6	1.4	–	–
$ 5000 – $ 6999	–	–	1.0	1.1
$ 7000 and over	2.5	2.3	–	–
$ 7000 – $ 9999	–	–	1.4	1.4
$10,000 – $14,999	–	–	1.8	1.9
$15,000 and over	–	–	2.4	2.5

1. *Source:* Department of Health, Education, and Welfare, *Health Statistics from the U.S. National Health Survey: Dental Care, Volume of Visits, United States, July 1957 – June 1959,* Series B-No. 15, Washington, D.C., April 1960, p. 17.

2. *Source: Department of Health, Edcuation, and Welfare, Volume of Dental Visits, United States, July 1963 – June 1964,* Public Health Service Publication No. 1000–Series 10, No. 23, Washington, D.C., October 1965, p. 18.

3. *Source:* Department of Health, Education, and Welfare, Public Health Service, *Monthly Vital Statistics Report: Health – Interview Survey – Provisional Data from the National Center for Health Statistics,* Vol. 18, No. 9, Supplement 2, December 18, 1969, pp. 6-7.

Source: Unpublished Data from the *Health Interview Survey,* National Center for Health Statistics, Public Health Service, Department of Health, Education, and Welfare, Rockville, Maryland.

Table 2-12. Percent Distribution of Dental Visits by Type of Service According to Family Income

Family Income		*Type of Service*						
	Fillings	Extractions	Cleaning/Examination	Straightening	Gum Treatment	Denture	Other	Total[3]
$ 0 – $3999								
1957-1958[1]	43.6	18.2	16.0	2.3	1.9	8.4	12.7	100.0
1963-1964[2]	31.4	26.0	27.2	3.3	4.6	18.0	–	100.0
$4000 – $6999								
1957-1958[1]	46.5	16.4	17.0	2.5	1.8	6.7	12.2	100.0
1963-1964[2]	40.4	18.2	29.6	3.7	3.5	12.0	–	100.0
$7000 and over								
1957-1958[1]	45.7	9.9	21.8	5.3	1.1	7.9	13.0	100.0
1963-1964[2]	38.1	10.1	39.4	7.7	3.4	12.7	–	100.0

1. *Source:* Department of Health, Education, and Welfare, *Health Statistics from the U.S. National Health Survey: Dental Care, Volume of Visits, United States, July 1957 – June 1959*, Series B-No. 15, Washington, D.C. April 1960, p. 28.

2. *Source:* Department of Health, Education, and Welfare, *Volume of Dental Visits, United States, July 1963 – June 1964* Public Health Service Publication No. 1000–Series 10, No. 23, Washington, D.C., October 1965, p. 32.

3. Figures may add to more than 100% because more than one type of service may be performed during a single visit.

Empirical Demand Studies

Several empirical analyses were conducted on the demand for dental care in an attempt to derive estimates of the price and income effect on dental expenditures and dental visits. The purpose of these analyses was to derive price and income elasticities that could then be used for forecasting purposes and later to help estimate the cost of several alternative national dental insurance plans (see Chapter 6). The empirical analyses used time series and cross sectional data as well as a single and multiple equation approach.

The results of the empirical demand studies are as follows.

Price. The reason for including a price variable was to determine the responsiveness of use of dental care (measured in terms of dental visits) to changes in its price. The effect of the price variable used in the analyses of the demand for dental visits per thousand population was highly significant (statistically) and its effect was in the expected direction. A 10 percent increase in price will lead to a 14.3 percent decrease in utilization, suggesting that the demand for dental care is price elastic. If better data become available, it would be useful to determine the price elasticity by income levels and by type of dental treatments demanded. Because of the unavailability of such data, only an aggregate measure of price elasticity was derived.[6]

Income. Income, as is generally known, is an important consideration in explaining expenditures on dental care. According to the results in all the regressions, the effect of income is positive and highly significant. With respect to the time series analyses, the magnitude is such that with an increase of 10 percent in income, expenditures on dental care will increase by more than 10 percent, to approximately 17 percent.[7]

The cross section results refer to differing expenditures by different income groups at a single point in time. Here it was found that a 10 percent increase in income increases *expenditures* on dental care by 10.3 percent in the analyses across states, and by 18.2 percent in the analyses across cities. When dental *visits* are used instead of expenditures, then a 10 percent increase in income increases the demand for visits by 15.5 percent, using the ADA data.[8] When expenditure data are used it should be kept in mind that an estimate of demand based on expenditures will probably exceed an estimate based on visits, if the rest of the data are comparable, because expenditures will reflect higher quality service or more expensive visits. The results of these empirical dental demand studies are presented in Appendix 2A.[9]

Fluoridation. In some of the empirical analyses it was possible to include a measure on the percent of the population using fluoridated water supplies. The fluoridation variable measures the change in dental expenditures resulting from the use of fluoridation. As seen from the regressions, which included a fluoridation variable, the effect of fluoridation is to cause a decrease in dental expenditure. Thus if we were to suppose that 100 percent of the population in a state used fluoridated water the effect would be a decrease of approximately $5.00 in per capita dental expenditures per year.[10]

Public expenditures per capita on dental health programs. Several of the empirical analyses included a variable that attempted to measure the effect on dental expenditures of public programs. The results were insignificant and were therefore excluded. It was thus not possible to show whether public expenditures serve to some extent as a substitute for private expenditures. The small amount spent (the average for all states being $.028 per capita) makes it difficult to isolate and measure its true effect.[11]

The findings of these empirical analyses are essentially threefold:

1. An increase in the price of dental care will lead to a proportionately greater decrease in the quantity of dental visits demanded. Similarly, the consequences of lowering the price of care through various forms of national dental insurance will lead to probably larger than expected increases in dental utilization.

2. An increase in income will lead to a proportionately larger increase in both dental expenditures and dental visits.

3. The results with respect to fluoridation are consistent with what other evidence on fluoridation has shown, namely, that an increase in the percent of the population using fluoridated water will result in very favorable cost savings in terms of decreases in dental use and expenditures.

Dental Insurance.

To date, dental insurance has not been a major economic factor influencing the demand for dental care. However, to accurately predict the demand for dental care it is necessary to be able to forecast the increase in dental insurance in the population as well as predict the effect that dental insurance will have on the demand for dental care. There is also a great deal of interest currently in dental insurance. It would therefore be useful at this point to provide a greater discussion of the determinants of the demand for dental insurance and of how insurance may affect the demand for dental care.

The Demand for Dental Insurance

There are several determinants of the demand for dental insurance; each of these will be discussed and then some empirical evidence examined in order to see how well the theory of demand for insurance confirms our expectations.

The theory of insurance suggests the type of services for which we would expect the purchase of insurance. The premium, which is the price of insurance, is composed of several factors: the administrative cost associated with claims processing, marketing, etc., and the "pure" premium, which is the actuarial value of the insurance policy. The actuarial value of a policy is related to the probability that an event will occur, multiplied by the expected loss if that event occurs. For example, if 100 people each have an equal chance of incurring an illness and the probability is 1:100 that someone would incur that illness, then each person has a 1 percent chance of being affected.

If the event occurs, and it requires a cost of $500.00, then if each person in the group of 100 paid $5.00, that amount would represent the pure premium of that risk. The size of that premium, therefore, is affected by the probability of the event's occurring and the size of the loss if it does occur. If the probability of a loss increases from 1 percent to 10 percent then each person will have to pay $50.00 to be insured. If the size of the loss increases to $1,000.00, then the premium would also rise. However, no insurance is sold purely at its actuarial value. Administrative costs must be added to it. The question, therefore, is how much over the actuarial value will a person be willing to pay for insurance?

The amount over the pure premium a person is willing to pay is related to several factors, such as how much of a risk he is willing to take himself. Not everyone buys insurance for everything. For some things people are willing to self-insure. This desire to self-insure is partly related to how risk-averse a person is and also to how large the possible loss might be if the unfortunate event occurs. Generally, the larger the possible loss the more likely one is to insure against it; similarly, we rarely observe people taking out insurance for events that are routine, predictable occurences for which the probability of the event's occurring is very high. Thus events that are not very likely to occur, but cost a great deal if they do occur, are more likely to be insured against than those events which are either a certainty (or similarly, events that have an extremely small probability of occurring) or cost relatively litte if they do occur.

That portion of the premium which is the administrative cost is likely to be larger if the probable loss is small than if it is a large loss. Therefore, a person might also be willing to insure against certain occurrences, which have a small probable loss, only if the amount over the actuarial value is relatively small; the larger the amount over the actuarial value, the more likely is he to self-insure. Further, it appears that administrative costs are larger for numerous small losses (claims) than they are for fewer very large losses.

If the number of claims are numerous, routine, and small in size, the administrative costs are presumably large in proportion to the actuarial value. A person purchasing "insurance" in this instance is really purchasing a budgeting system for himself. This type of purchase is not a method of insuring against risks, but merely one of *prepaying* his expected expenses. Prepayment is thus a time payment device rather than a method of spreading risk. In discussions of the demand for insurance it is important to distinguish between prepayment and insurance, since the determinants of demand for each are different; if we wish to predict the growth in dental coverage it is necessary to ascertain whether dental coverage is more reflective of prepayment than insurance.

Our theory of insurance, therefore, would lead us to predict that the demand for a particular form of insurance would depend on the probability of an event's occuring, the size of the loss if it does occur, and the amount above the pure premium one must pay for that insurance. The "price" of insurance may thus be considered the amount over the pure premium a person must pay. Other things held constant, the lower the price, the greater the demand for insurance.

Another factor that will affect the demand for insurance is family income. The effect of increased income is such that with more money a family can buy more of everything and, second, health insurance has become an important fringe benefit. With higher incomes (hence a higher tax bracket) if the employer buys the insurance for an employee, more can be purchased than if the employee received an equivalent amount of money in cash, paid taxes on it, and then bought insurance. It is also possible that with increased incomes there will be a tendency for the demand for dental insurance to decrease because high income families would be more likely to cover the possible loss themselves. The likelihood of self-insurance would be greater given the relatively low level of dental care costs in relation to the higher incomes.

When we apply the above theory of insurance to the health field we observe that insurance is more likely to be purchased in those cases where the probability of occurrence is small but the size of the loss is large; that is, hospitalization insurance is more likely to be purchased than is dental insurance. Further, with increased incomes, health insurance has become an important fringe benefit for many unions. We would expect that dental insurance is unlikely to be purchased except as a fringe benefit.

The above discussion assumed that there was no "moral hazard" involved in the purchase of insurance. If a person with insurance can affect the size of the loss, then the purchase of such insurance is less likely, unless certain limits and controls are imposed. The reason for this is that the actuarial value of the insurance is likely to be greater if people can increase their use. Consider for example two groups of users: "high users" who buy insurance because they expect to use more dental care the value of which is more than the premium they pay for the insurance; and "low users," who purchase insurance without any expectation of higher use. If the low users have to choose between self-insuring against the loss and selecting a premium higher than the actuarial value they would be willing to pay (because once a person pays the premium his use will increase), then they might decide to self-insure. The premium would be more attractive to these persons if it were lower; this could be achieved if copayments such as deductibles and coinsurance, were included. Therefore when "moral hazard" exists, persons would be more apt to purchase insurance if they could bear part of the expense in the form of copayments. We would expect this to be the case with dental insurance. The premium for dental insurance (or prepayment) would be larger than a person might be willing to pay, since everyone else insured will cause the premium to be greater than the person expected it to be. Copayments would reduce use and the premium.[12]

There are several additional factors which will affect the premium a person must pay, hence his demand for insurance; one of these is whether or not the person buying insurance is a member of a group or is just an individual purchaser. There are economies to administering group claims compared to administering the same number of individual claims. This difference in cost would be reflected in the premium a person must pay. Therefore group insurance would be preferred to nongroup insurance by individuals because, ceteris paribus, it is lower in price.

A major factor affecting the size of the premium is the method used to reimburse the provider (the dentist) for his services. Some methods of provider payment would presumably result in lower price and quantity of dental service than other methods, and this would be reflected in lower premiums. The main bases of provider reimbursement are fee-for-service and capitation, and these can be paid for on an indemnity basis or as a service benefit. Each of these will be briefly discussed together with its hypothesized effects.

Fee-for-service provides an incentive on the part of the provider for increased use and more frequent call backs. The effect of capitation reimbursement may be just the opposite; the provider has an incentive to reduce the number of visits (and increase the number of patients). The effectiveness of either approach has not been clearly demonstrated and depends on the ability of the consumer to choose between these two approaches based on price and quality of care. To date, such information is not made available to the consumer.

These alternative systems of reimbursement could coexist with one another in the same community, but the consumer would obviously benefit if he were provided more information with which to make choices. Traditionally, the health field has considered it "unethical" to provide the consumer with the necessary information with which to make decisions. The effect of more information on prices and quality of dental care should be examined. Alternative hypotheses regarding the lack of information may relate to the impact of greater information on the consumer, as well as the impact on provider behavior and performance.

Under indemnity reimbursement a patient will receive payment from the insurance company and reimburse the provider. The indemnity, in most cases, is not for the same amount as the provider's bill. The critics of indemnities, primarily with regard to large bills such as hospital utilization, suggest that the indemnities will be too little to reimburse the provider for the episode of illness. Proponents of indemnities suggest that it serves as an incentive to the consumer to shop around (be more price conscious) and not to overuse services.

Service benefits, on the other hand, are generally reimbursement in full for the service provided, and most likely go from the insurance company directly to the provider upon submission of a bill. The proponents of service benefits would suggest that a patient need not worry about having to pay for part of the bill, while the critics of service benefits point to the incentive on the part of providers to raise their prices since they will be reimbursed in full; the patient also lacks any incentive under service benefit payment to seek out lower priced providers.

The above discussion on provider payment has been very brief. It is a very important area of concern in financing health care and could have a substantial impact on prices, quantity, and quality. To date, many of the issues involved in provider payment are made complex because there is a mixture of value judgments regarding how much care a consumer should receive as well as the ability of the consumer to discriminate between variations in prices and the quality of the service. There is also a lack of empirical knowledge concerning the effects of different methods of payment. Certainly more experimentation should be undertaken in this area, together with a proper evaluation of the results.[13]

In summary, the factors that affect a person's demand for dental insurance are the price (the amount above the pure premium that he must pay for that insurance), and his income, particularly because of the tax deductibility of fringe benefits. The price of the insurance is likely to be higher in cases of higher administrative cost in relation to the pure premium, of the existence of "moral hazard," of individual rather than group purchase of insurance, and when the provider is reimbursed on a fee-for-service payment under a service benefit. The higher the price of dental insurance, the less likely is its growth in the population. Offsetting such likely "high" prices for dental insurance, however, is the growth in incomes, hence increased use of fringe benefits. To date, the growth in dental insurance, shown in Table 2-13, has been slow. Only .2 percent of the U.S. population had some form of dental insurance in 1950; this figure had grown to 6.3 percent by 1970.

Table 2-13. Percent of Population Having Some Form of Dental Insurance, 1950-1970

Year	Percent Covered
1970	6.3
1969	4.7
1968	3.5
1967	2.0
1966	1.6
1965	1.0
1960	0.4
1950	0.2

Source: Division of Dental Health, U.S. Department of Health, Education, and Welfare

While it appears that the income effect will cause continued growth, particularly in unionized industries, it does not appear likely that large segments of the population will be covered in the next ten years unless a sizeable federal program brings this about. The growth in dental insurance would be greater if it were to limit coverage to those instances where it is more of an insurable risk — that is, where moral hazard is low and the potential treatment costs are high. This would suggest that dental insurance should cover only those treatment costs such as emergency care, birth defects in children, and perhaps peridontal diseases.

Dental Insurance as a Factor Affecting Demand
for Dental Care

The existence of dental insurance is expected to affect people's demand for dental care because it removes (all or in part) the financial barriers to seeking dental care. The impact of dental insurance on demand for care is important to determine if we are to propose extensions of this insurance to various population groups in society. Unless its probable impact is known, it will not only be difficult to forecast the costs of such programs but, more important, we will not know whether the provision of dental insurance will achieve certain social goals by extending it to those who need dental care. Dental insurance comes in many sizes and packages. The particular method of coverage and type of payment used will affect the demand for care as well as having different effects on the overall cost of dental care.

The general types of coverages may vary from payment in full for all a person's dental care to the imposition of various combinations of deductibles, copayment features, to limits on the extent of coverage, and to whether or not it is treatment specific. The basic reason for having limits of any type is that there is a problem of what is known in the insurance literature as "moral hazard" associated with dental care — that is, the insured can affect the size of the loss.[14] (As discussed earlier, the existence of moral hazard also affects the demand for dental insurance.) Dental insurance is different from life insurance or fire insurance in that it is generally assumed that life and fire insurance are mechanisms which can be used to share the risk of possible large losses, and that the person insuring against those risks is not more likely to incur those risks once he is insured. Insurance for dental care, however, may influence not only when a person uses dental care, but also how much of it he uses. In order both to limit use and develop actuarially fair premiums, various limits and controls are usually included in dental insurance plans.

A discussion of several of these limits and controls in dental insurance and their expected effects follows.

Deductibles. A deductible provision means that a family (or person) must pay a certain amount of money before he is entitled to receive benefits or be reimbursed for his dental care. The deductible may or may not be related to specific treatments. The deductible may be set low or high for different reasons. If it is low, then it is believed that only some minor forms of care should be discouraged, whereas a high deductible suggests that a family should pay for its own care, except for catastrophic illnesses. It is important to be explicit regarding one's objectives if deductibles (and other limits) are imposed so that the effect is what was intended. The effect of deductibles on demand for care will also vary according to whether or not the deductible is related to a person's income. For example, a low deductible for everyone regardless of income will discourage dental care for the poor and have little effect on use by the higher income families.

What can be predicted about the use of the deductible in dental insurance? If it is set low in relation to per capita expenditures for dental care, then it will not limit utilization for those whose expenditures exceed (or expect to exceed) the deductible; while for those persons whose dental care expenditures are below that amount (generally the poor) it will not encourage greater use.[a] Thus once the deductible has been paid, and there are no additional financial barriers past the deductible such as copayments, then the existence of a deductible is unlikely to affect utilization of services for the above reasons.

The size of the deductible in relation to a family's expected expenditures for dental care will determine whether it either has no effect on use (for those whose expenditures are less than the deductible) or whether it no longer serves as a limit on use (for those families who expect to exceed the deductible). Low income persons would thus be more adversely affected by a deductible. In order to determine the impact of the deductible in terms of its effect on families, classified by income levels and other determinants of demand such as age, as well as the probable cost of a deductible type of program, it is necessary to look at the distribution of expenditures for dental care by family characteristics.

Figure 2-1 shows the distribution of dental expenditures among families with different incomes. According to this diagram we can visualize what the expected effect of a certain deductible and of different size deductibles is likely to be. As the size of the deductible is increased, fewer families would benefit. However, families who would benefit most from a given size deductible would be those families with predominantly higher incomes, since proportionately more of the higher income families have expenditures that exceed the deductible. If a deductible were to be imposed, it would lead to more equitable utilization if it were related to income level.

Coinsurance. When a person is reimbursed for a portion of his dental expenditures, the coinsurance will affect his use of dental services just as would a reduction in the price of those services. For example, if a coinsurance provision requires the person to pay only 80 percent of the price of dental care, then this is equivalent to a 20 percent reduction in the price to him. The impact of such coinsurance on the demand for dental care will depend upon the "price elasticity" of demand for such care, i.e., how responsive the use of dental services is to changes in its price.

---

[a] It is conceivable that people who would not purchase as much as the deductible without a deductible, might in fact purchase more than the deductible, given a deductible. The extent to which consumer preferences would change would depend upon the size of the deductible in relation to their current expenditures on dental care and the utility they receive from additional amounts of dental care compared to their utility to be received from other purchases with those same additional funds.

Figure 2-1. Distribution of Dental Expenses by Families with Different Incomes, 1958

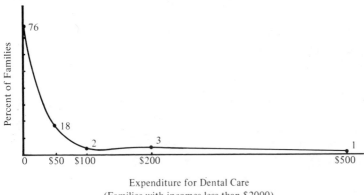

Expenditure for Dental Care
(Families with incomes less than $2000)

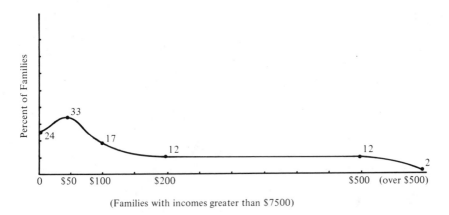

(Families with incomes greater than $7500)

Source: O.W. Anderson, P. Collette and J.J. Feldman, *Family Expenditure Patterns for Personal Health Services,* Health Information Foundation Research Series no. 14, p. 61.

A diagram might serve to clarify the effect of coinsurance on demand for care. Figure 2-2 shows the relationship between price of dental care and quantity of dental care demanded, all other determinants of demand being held constant. If the price were P_1 then according to the relationship between price and quantity demanded, the quantity demanded will be Q_1. If insurance for dental care were provided and it included a coinsurance feature, then the person would have to pay a portion of the price. The new price to be paid by the enrollee will be P_2, which is, for example, 80 percent of P_1. (The third party will pay the difference, P_1-P_2.) The increased use of dental services as a result of the lower price will be Q_2. The extent of increased demand as a result of a coinsurance feature will depend on the size of the coinsurance, the price elasticity of demand, and a family's income. As long as there is some responsiveness of

48

Figure 2-2. The Effect of Co-Insurance on the Demand for Dental Care

Quantity of Dental Care Used in a Year

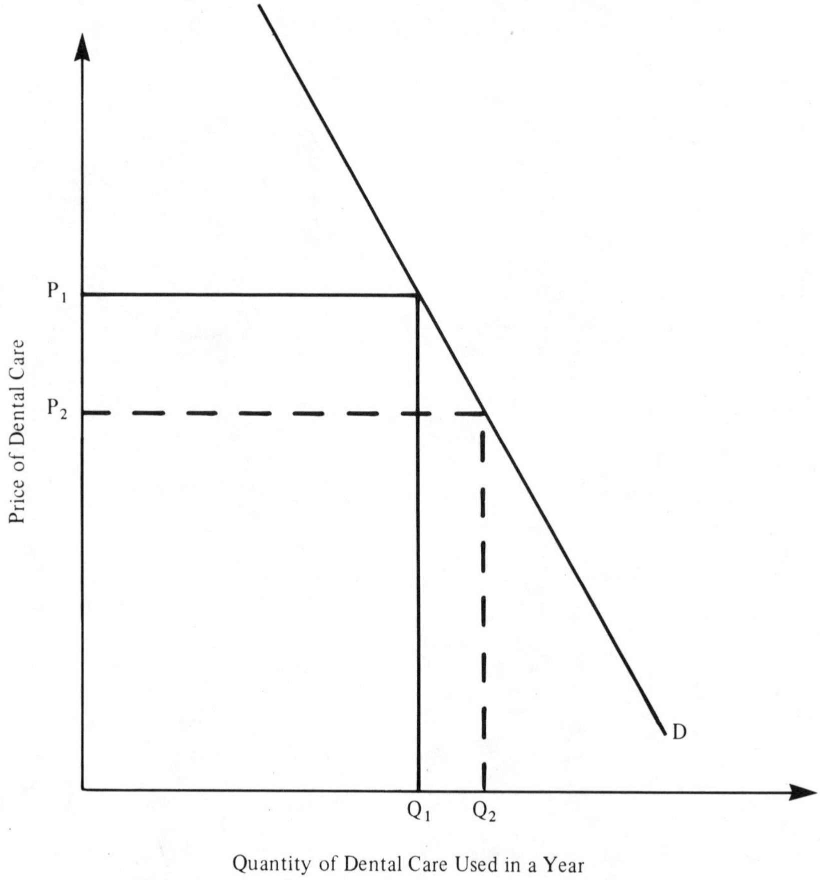

demand to price, then a coinsurance feature in an insurance plan will limit use of services.

For a specific level of coinsurance, the actual price the consumer will pay for dental care and his actual consumption will depend upon the elasticities of the demand and supply of dental care. The more elastic they both are, the greater the consumption and the less the rise in price to the consumer.

For example, according to Figure 2-3, the consumer's original demand curve is D_1. With a coinsurance provision (for simplicity, it is assumed to be 50 percent, with the remainder to be paid by the government) there will be a shift in the demand for dental care to D_2, which represent the amount that both the consumers and the government will pay for dental care. (Thus every point of D_2 represents a doubling of the price for a given quantity over D_1, since it is a 50 percent coinsurance program). Because the new demand curve intersects the supply curve at a higher price than previously, there will be a new equilibrium

Figure 2-3. The Effect of Co-Insurance on the Aggregate Demand for Dental Care

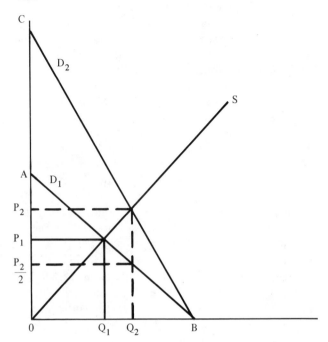

price and quantity for dental care, which will be P_2 and Q_2. (Q_2 is thus the only level of quantity at which the public pays one-half the price of dental care $\left(\dfrac{P_2}{2}\right)$ and is also an equilibrium position. Thus the price the consumer will pay with a 50 percent coinsurance is greater than 50 percent of the original market price $\left(\dfrac{P_1}{2}\right)$. The introduction of a copayment feature does not mean that the consumer's price will be a similar percent of the original market price. Nor does it mean that the amount of care used will increase by that same proportion. The greater the coinsurance paid for by the government (or other third party) the greater will be the consumer's use of dental services, but the actual price he must pay and the amount he will actually consume depends upon the elasticity of both demand and supply.

Lower income families, with presumably a lower price elasticity of demand, will not increase their utilization by as much as higher income families for a given decrease in price. Again, the objective of coinsurance features in relation to income levels in any national dental insurance program should be made explicit if dental services are to be used by the persons intended and to the degree to which it was intended.

Other Limits and Controls

Besides deductibles and coinsurance there are other methods used to limit and control use or to make a dental insurance plan financially solvent. These methods are basically modifications of the deductible and coinsurance features; for example, an upper limit may be placed on the amount of dental services to be reimbursed, which is equivalent to setting the coinsurance rate equal to the market price as that limit is reached. If the type of dental care used beyond this upper limit is necessary, then such limits will have the effect of decreasing the use of such services, particularly by the lower income families. If such care is required, then the effect of this upper limit will be to cause the patients to seek out the lowest cost providers, and/or lowest quality providers. The theory behind insurance is that it should cover the very large expenses of a few persons; this is similar to risk sharing. Insurance coverage that provides coverage up to a maximum for medically needed services goes contrary to the basic idea of insurance. It is with respect to such large expenditures for relatively few persons that insurance is particularly important if it is not to be a financial hardship. Further, the premiums for this portion of the bill are relatively inexpensive.

Other types of insurance limits exclude certain forms of treatment from coverage. The considerations involved in this type of coverage should be to cover those forms of care that are medically required and to exclude others where more discretionary use exists among the patients, or which are used predominantly by higher income families. Dental insurance can, and does, use a variety of such types of limits and controls. They can be used singly or in combination with one another, e.g., deductibles and coinsurance.

Another method commonly used in some dental insurance plans is to impose a minimum time limit for which a person can join a dental plan, such as for three years. Without time limits, it is feared that a person would remain a member only as long as is necessary to have all the dental work he wants. Under such a circumstance the person's premium would not reflect the costs he incurs, and therefore the dental plan would not be financially viable, or other members would be required to subsidize the person's use. As an alternative to minimum times for membership, some plans require substantial payments by the individual to reach a specified level of dental health before he can receive benefits from the dental plan.[15]

To reemphasize, the basic reason behind most of the variations in types of coverage under dental insurance plans is because of the problem of "moral hazard" – that is, the insured can affect the size of the loss. If it were not for the fact that the insured can affect his use of such services, then there would be little need for controls or limits.[16]

Summary of the Demand for Dental Care

Expenditures on dental care, regardless of the source used, have been increasing over time. In order to both be able to understand the reasons for this increase and be able to forecast trends in expenditures more accurately, it is necessary to separate expenditures into its component parts. When adjusted for population, per capita expenditures have increased because of increases in both the price of dental care and in visits per capita. An examination of the reasons for increases in price and quantity therefore necessitates an examination of both the supply and demand for dental care. In this chapter on demand, the factors affecting demand were categorized into need, attitudes toward dental care, and economic variables. Increases in need would result in increases in demand, holding constant both attitude and economic factors. The use of dental symptoms and age as measures of need were examined. Fluoridation was also discussed because of its influence in decreasing need for certain types of dental treatments. The number of persons using fluoridated water has increased greatly in the past ten years but there is a large percent of the population still without fluoridated water supplies. It would appear that a continuation of trends toward fluoridation (as well as other preventive measures) would result in large decreases in need, and hence lower future demands for some forms of dental care.

However, need alone does not explain all the variations in demand for dental care, as seen by the data on dental symptoms and age. Other factors are also important in explaining differences in demand. Using data on education of the head of the household as a measure of attitudes, we observe that differences in education, within income class, are also significant. Attitudes are changed slowly, however, therefore if it is desired to change the demand for dental care, then in addition to preventive measures as fluoridation one must be able to influence the economic factors affecting demand. The major economic variables are the consumer's income and the price he must pay for the care. Although income has been shown to be important in many surveys, it is necessary to estimate the net effect that income has on dental use and expenditures. According to the empirical analyses and the review of other studies, it was determined that if income increases by 10 percent, expenditures and use of dental care will increase by a proportionally larger amount, approximately 15 percent.

The implications of this finding is that past increases in personal incomes have led to large increases in the demand for care and that this will continue into the future. This projected increase in demand may express itself in two ways. With higher incomes, more may be spent directly on dental care. Alternatively, and in conjunction with the above, there may be an increase in demand for fringe benefits providing prepaid dental care. This is because employers' contributions for the payment of health insurance premiums do not constitute taxable income to the recipients. Thus there is a tax incentive at higher income levels for increased indirect dental expenditures in the form of increased employer contributions.

The increased demand for dental care that comes with higher incomes will cause a rise in dental care prices. Prices will rise because the supply of dental care is not very responsive to changes in price of dental care in the short run, due to length of time required to train new dentists and build new dental schools.

The effect of higher prices for dental care will, according to the empirical analyses, cause proportionately greater decreases in the quantity of dental visits demanded. Previous studies on demand and use of dental care have excluded the influence of price on utilization. The problem caused by this is that the effects attributed to other factors such as income, age, etc., might also include the effects of higher dental prices. The effects of these other, nonprice factors would thus tend to be inaccurately estimated.

The impact of the growth in dental insurance on demand for dental care would depend to an important degree on which benefits are covered and the price elasticity of demand for the covered services. A fruitful area for research would be to develop accurate estimates of the price elasticity of demand by treatment category as well as within each income classification.

As an illustration of the usefulness of price and income elasticities in the analysis of the demand for dental care, an attempt was made to explain the increase in visits per capita over time. From 1955 to 1970, total visits for dental care (using ADA data) increased 48 percent. Population also increased over that time so in terms of visits per capita the increase was 20 percent. Over that same time period personal income per capita rose 77 percent and the price of dental care increased 46 percent. Thus the effect of rising incomes was to increase the demand for dental care by 131 percent (77 percent multiplied by an income elasticity of 1.71). Over that period, the rise in dental prices caused a decrease in demand of 65 percent (46 percent multiplied by the price elasticity of -1.43). Since visits per capita increased by 20 percent, the difference is a decrease in demand by other factors over that period of 46 percent ($131 - 65 = 66 - 20 = 46$). This decrease in visits per capita of 46 percent might have been caused by a number of factors, fluoridation probably being the major one.[b]

In conclusion, given a continued rise in income accompanied by increased demand for dental care, and given the unresponsiveness of supply to rising prices, we would hypothesize that the price of dental care will continue to increase in the future. This will further limit the amount of dental care that the lowest income groups can afford. With an increase in demand, the amount by which price will change will be affected by how supply will respond to the increase in demand. Therefore, we turn our attention next to the determinants of the supply of dental care, including its distribution and use in order to be able to forecast the effect on supply of alternative policies that propose to increase it.

---

[b]In Chapter 5 an econometric model is used to make forecasts of dental prices, visits, expenditures, and dental incomes for 1975 based on several assumptions regarding population and personal incomes at that time.

Appendix 2A. Empirical Analyses of the Demand for Dental Care

1. Time Series Analyses of Per Capita Expenditures on Dental Care, 1929-1970

	Constant Term	Per Capita Income	R^2	N
(Year to Year Changes)	.093	.0048 (.0007)	.52	41
(In Logarithms)	−5.394	1.022 (.031)	.98	42

2. Cross Section Analyses of Family Expenditure on Dental Care, 1960-1961
(Data for 38 United States cities)

	Constant Term	Family Income	Use of Fluoride Water	R^2	N
	−28.34	+.013[b] (.002)	−5.24[a] (3.63)	.61	38
(In Logarithms)	− 5.28	+1.82[b] (.23)	—	.64	38

3. Cross Section Analyses of Per Capita Expenditure on Dental Care by States

	Year	Constant Term	Per Capita Income	Percent of Population Using Flouride Water	R^2
	1960	− .4781	+.0060[b] (.0012)	−.0433[b] (.0292)	.43
(In Logarithms)	1960	−2.9120	+1.222[b] (.227)	−.0932[a] (.0698)	.48
	1967	.8409	.0047[a] (.0009)	−.0506[b] (.0268)	.49
(In Logarithms)	1967	−5.3417	1.032[a] (.184)	−.1095[b] (.0463)	.57

[a]Significant at the .01 level.

[b]Significant at the .05 level.

Appendix 2B. Data Sources for Empirical Dental Demand Analyses

1. *Time Series*

Personal consumption expenditures on dental care: from U.S. Department of Commerce, Office of Business Economics: *National Income, 1954 ed.; U.S. Income and Output, 1958 ed.; Survey of Current Business,* July 1961, 1964, and 1968. From Social Security Administration, Office of Research and Statistics: Barbara Cooper and Nancy Worthington, National Health Expenditures, Calendar Years 1929-70, Research and Statistics Note No. 1, 1972.

Disposable income: from U.S. Bureau of the Census, *Historical Statistics of the United States* and *Statistical Abstract of the United States* (various editions).

Population of the United States: from U.S. Bureau of Census, *Statistical Abstract of the United States,* 1971, p. 5.

2. *Cross Section Analyses by States*

Per Capita Expenditures on Dental Care, by State: from Social Security Administration, Office of Research and Statistics: Louis S. Reed, *Per Capita Expenditures for Hospital Care and for the Services of Physicians and Dentists, by Region and State,* Research and Statistics Note No. 18, 1964; Louis S. Reed and Willine Carr, *Per Capita Expenditures for Hospital Care, the Services of Physicians and Dentists, and Private Insurance by Region and State, 1966,* Research and Statistics Note No. 13, 1969.

Per Capita Personal Income, by State: U.S. Department of Commerce, Office of Business Economics, *Personal Income by States, a Supplement to the Survey of Current Business, and Survey of Current Business,* August 1964; U.S. Bureau of the Census, *Statistical Abstract of the United States, 1969.*

Percent on Population Using Fluoridated Water, by State: U.S. Department of Health, Education, and Welfare, Division of Public Health and Resources, *Fluoridation Census 1965.* (A time lage of 3 to 4 years is necessary before a fluoridated water supply begins to have beneficial effects on the dental health of its subscribers; this time lag is properly reflected in the 1967 regressions but not in the 1960 regressions.)

3. *Cross Section Analyses by Cities*

Family Income, 1960-1961: U.S. Department of Labor, Bureau of Labor Statistics, *Survey of Consumer Expenditures,* Special City Tabulations.

Family Expenditure on Dental Care, 1960-1961: ibid.

Number of Years a City Has Used Fluoridated Water: U.S. Department of Health, Education, and Welfare, Division of Public Health and Resources, *Fluoridation Census 1965* (data as of 1961).

The Supply of Dental Care

Distribution and Use of Dental Services

The distribution of dentists among states varies greatly. Those states with the highest dentist-population ratios have up to three times as many dentists per thousand population as those states with the lowest dentist-population ratios. A comparison of states with the highest and lowest ratios is shown in Table 3-1. Generally, rural areas tend to have lower dentist-population ratios and these tend

Table 3-1. Geographic Disparities in the Number of Dentists, 1969

State	Population per Dentist
New York	1,232
Oregon	1,282
Massachusetts	1,363
Minnesota	1,385
Washington	1,427
Arkansas	3,041
North Carolina	3,045
Alabama	3,100
South Carolina	3,625
Mississippi	3,685

Source: Distribution of Dentists in the United States by State, Region, District, and County, American Dental Association, 1970, p. 4.

to be the poorer areas. Within urban areas dentists also have a tendency to be distributed according to the incomes of the different areas. The low income areas tend to have very low dentist-population ratios, and the middle and upper class areas much higher ratios.

The problem of achieving a more "equitable" distribution of dental resources has concerned people who wish to increase the level of oral health in poor and rural areas. In order to examine alternative public policies with regard to a more equitable distribution of dental care, the causes of such an uneven distribution must be determined.

Hypotheses Regarding the Distribution of Dentists

The distribution, use, and availability of dental care is basically a microcosm of the national problem, with some modifications. The financing issues involved are therefore also similar. On a national level it has been said that differences in use of dental services between population groups are related to differences in demand for care as well as supply conditions. Persons having higher incomes (other things being equal among the groups) would have a greater demand for dental care. And if the conditions of supply were similar for groups, we would expect to observe higher levels of use for those persons with higher incomes. This analysis of the problem of uneven distribution suggests that we should examine differences in demand for dental care as a prime determinant of differences in use. Further, public policy that seeks to increase use in low use areas should examine the potential of stimulating the demand for such care.

The assumption underlying this approach is that supply would respond to increased demand for care. If, however, the market for dental services is not working as described above, then merely increasing demand for care may not achieve the policy goals of increased use. The empirical question therefore is the extent to which the number of dentists responds to changes in demand.

An inadequate supply response to increased demand may occur if there are barriers preventing this response. It is important therefore both to determine whether (and the extent to which) supply responds to such increased demands, and/or to remove or reduce barriers that inhibit a greater supply response. The policy implications regarding the uneven use of dental services would also be applicable on a national level. Barriers would affect increases in the supply of dental manpower over time rather than interstate mobility of dentists.

Empirical Analyses of the Distribution of Dentists

Several studies have attempted to determine the reasons for the uneven distribution of dentists among states.[1] In the study by Benham, Maurizi, and Reder, an examination was made to determine how the distribution of dentists between states was influenced by the demand for dental services, the locational preferences of dentists, and the barriers to migration.

The analyses on distribution of dentists among states was conducted for the time periods 1930, 1940, 1950 and 1960. The statistical analysis also tried to explain the change in dentists between states for each of the above time periods, i.e., 1930-1940, 1940-1950, and 1950-1960. The variables used to explain the number of dentists and the change in the number of dentists within a state were population, personal income in that state, volume of training facilities, degree of urbanization, average income of dentists in that state, and the percentage of applicants for licensure who fail examinations (as a measure of barriers to entry).

The statistical results, using multiple regression analysis, were all highly significant (statistically) and were able to explain a large part of the interstate variations in dentists, dentist-population ratios, and changes in dentists over time. Since there were an extensive number of regression analyses, they will not be reproduced here; however, their findings on the distribution of dentists with respect to the above variables will be discussed.

Demands for dental services. Two variables were employed as determinants of demand: population and per capita income within a state. Both variables were statistically significant and were found to be major determinants of the number of dentists within a state. The implication of the findings of this analysis with respect to the two demand factors is that the number and changes in dentists within a state are highly responsive to demand forces; market forces are very important in directing the flow of dentists.

Barriers to migration. Failure rates on licensing examinations in a state was used as a measure of limiting the entry of dentists to a state. The licensing examination given by a state is the same for all dentists wishing to practice in that state, regardless of where in the United States the dentist attended school. However, state examinations may differ since they may concentrate on some technique more than others and in this fashion graduates of schools from that state would have an advantage in taking the exam.

Since there is little reciprocity between states it has been alleged that the licensing exam in a given state has been used to reduce the number of dentists who wish to practice in a state. This variable proved to be statistically significant, indicating that increased failure rates decreased the number of dentists migrating into a state. When failure rates are used in a multivariate analysis of dental incomes in a state we observe that the higher the failure rates on examinations (other factors held constant) the greater the dental incomes. The implication of the correlation of failure rates, number of dentists, and dental incomes is that examination failure is used as a barrier to the flow of dentists into areas where there are higher dental incomes. Failure rates in dental examinations might thus be considered a means of maintaining dental incomes rather than maintaining quality within a state.

Locational preferences of dentists. At least two variables were used in the analyses to measure locational preferences of dentists: the number of dentists' training facilities in a state, and the degree of urbanization of a state. The results were not entirely satisfactory; the significance of these variables were not stable for different time periods and the authors concluded that the inconclusiveness of these variables was probably a result of statistical problems with the data.

To summarize the locational determinants of dentists, it was found that demand forces have a strong influence on the number of dentists practicing within a state. Increased demands for dental care, hence higher dental incomes, would cause in-migration of dentists to a state. This supply responsiveness to increased demand more than outweighs any locational preferences of dentists. Unfortunately, an impediment to this supply response has been the manner in which licensing examinations have been administered. The authors of the study suggest that "changes in the policies and quite possibly in the manner of selecting members of state examining boards, would be in the public interest."[2]

Limiting entry to a state in order to maintain dental incomes inhibits the adjustment process of changes in demand and supply from occuring. It also results in higher costs of dental care and a smaller availability of such care, as well as imposing greater costs of educating prospective dentists. If there were greater interstate mobility of dentists, then the dental school in which a student enrolls need not be in the region where he wished to practice. Since there are economies of scale in the production of dental students (see Chapter 4, Table 4-6) then fewer states would need dental schools, with the existing schools each becoming larger and achieving lower per student costs.[3]

Subsidizing the In-Migration of Dentists to a State

If it is desirable to increase the use of dental care by those in low income or rural areas, one policy for achieving this objective is to increase the demand for care in those areas. Further, if it is desired for various reasons to increase the supply of dental care available, this may be achieved by increasing the use of auxiliaries or more highly trained assistants rather than merely increasing the number of dentits. If, however, we want to increase the dentist-population ratio in a state, several alternatives exist. A state could subsidize the construction of a dental school and its operating costs in the hope that the graduates would remain in the state after graduation (or use forgiveness loans if they were to practice in specified areas for a maximum period of time). Alternatively, the state could achieve the same increase in the number of dentists in a shorter period of time by subsidizing out-of-state dentists to relocate in the state or in a particular area.

It is important to specify the objective of proposals in order to develop alternatives and make comparisons between them. If the priorities of a state were to achieve an increase in the oral health status of specific population groups, then one subobjective with regard to this overall objective *might* be to increase the dentist-population ratio of that state. In meeting this subobjective, the state should compare the cost of subsidizing nonstate dentists to relocate in the state as against construction and operating subsidies for additional dental school capacity. Based upon preliminary calculations, it would appear that states having lower dentist-population ratios would find it far less expensive (it would cost approximately one-fourth to one-half as much) and a more speedy solution to subsidize dentists to relocate rather than to produce additional dentists themselves.[a]

Comments on the Uneven Distribution of Dentists

This section on distribution of dentists has been brief because it is believed to be similar in both analyses and policy alternatives to the more general problem of

----

[a]These calculations and their underlying assumptions are discussed more completely in Appendix 3A.

The purpose of the above analysis is to illustrate the costs of two choices for increasing the supply of dentists in a state. The costs of each of these choices would obviously be affected by the number of states attempting to subsidize in-migration of dentists and the number of dentists they wished to attract. The number of dentists remaining in a state as a result of additional dental school capacity would also depend upon the amount by which dental school capacity is increased.

differences in use of dental care by different population groups. The similarity of the distribution problem to that of differences between users of dental care on a national level is that use is importantly affected by demand factors – i.e., that the supply of dental services responds to increases in demand to the extent that there are few barriers to interstate mobility or barriers to entering the profession. Dentists are but one input into the production of dental services; therefore, increases in the supply of dental services to these areas can also be achieved through increased use of auxiliaries either in conjunction with dentists or on their own with additional training.

Since the demand for dental care is highly responsive to increased consumer income, perhaps greater reliance should be placed on stimulating the demand on behalf of those who need more care. Policies that increase the supply of dentists in a state do not necessarily mean that those who need the services will receive them; they may still be unable to afford or unwilling to purchase such services.

Demand stimulating policies may at times be supplemented by additional programs. In situations where there are low population densities, or in urban areas where the poor must travel greater distances to receive dental care, the problem of accessibility (high travel cost measured in either lost time or actual out-of-pocket expense) may act as much a deterrent to use of dental services as inability to pay. In such cases alternatives for decreasing these travel costs should be considered. On the demand side this may mean paying out-of-pocket travel costs or, considering a supply alternative, it may mean achieving greater flexibility in using the dentist or his auxiliaries in relation to the population to be served (e.g., mobile dental vehicles). If the problem is accessibility, either of these might be a less expensive alternative than simply subsidizing more dentists to locate in sparcely populated areas.

In order to maximize the use of dental services with a given budget (measured in either dollars or personnel) for persons living in areas where use and distribution of dental services are low, consideration must be given to alternative means of achieving this goal.

Supply of Dental Care

Dental services can be financed through the demand side by increasing the demand for such services, or through the supply side by increasing the availability of supply and supply factors. The effectiveness of financing programs on the demand side will depend on the supply of dental care. That is, if the supply of dentists does not increase, then increased demand would cause large increases in price, only small increases in dental utilization (primarily from existing dentists), and the goals of the financing program will probably not be attained. If, however, the supply response (i.e., increases in the number of dentists) is rapid and large with an increase in demand then the expenditures involved in a financing program will result in large increases in dental care utilization. Since prices, utilization, and expenditures are all affected by conditions of supply it becomes important to ascertain the determinants of the supply of dental care. In this way we can predict what the likely supply response will be in the future, hence the effect that various demand financing programs will have. We are also interested in analyzing the supply side of the dental market because some large financing programs are directed toward increasing the supply of dental care services. Unless we can anticipate the effect of such programs for financing supply, we may not achieve our goals, and more importantly, we will lose the opportunity for comparing alternative approaches for achieving our goals.

In addition to being able to anticipate the effects of different financing programs there is another reason for investigating the supply side of the dental market: to determine how efficiently the current system of delivery is performing, compared to proposed changes that may be made in that system. (By efficiency in production we mean either that the quantity and quality of dental care can not be greater with the same level of expenditure, or that the same quantity or quality can not be achieved at a lower cost.) Further, the adoption or implementation of various proposed changes regarding the supply of services or manpower is determined by the conditions that currently structure the supply side.

The reasons, then, for an examination of the determinants of supply of dental services are to predict the effects of financing programs on the demand side, to be able to anticipate the supply response of proposed programs for increasing the supply of dental care, and to be able to make some tentative comments on the economic efficiency of the dental market.

A Model of the Supply of Dental Services

As a means of outlining the discussion to follow, a framework is presented that should also serve as a basis for the type of data to be collected and for the economic research to be conducted in this area. The supply of dental care has several interrelated levels. Since this book has been primarily concerned with the market for dental care services and not oral health status per se, we will take as our broadest and first level the supply of dental services. Our concern should be with oral health status, where the provision and use of dental services is but one way of affecting oral health. Financing objectives should therefore be evaluated in terms of affecting the oral health status of particular groups. In this regard the financing of dental services is but one way of achieving our goals and should be evaluated with regard to these alternatives. The emphasis on supply of dental services occurs because it is at this level that there is a great deal of concern and, currently, financing programs.

The supply of dental services can be produced in different settings, with different combinations of dental personnel and equipment. The supply of these inputs — dentists, auxiliary personnel, capital, and equipment — comprise the next level in the supply of services. The supply of specific inputs are each determined by a number of factors. If we wish to increase the supply of dental services, this can be achieved by increasing one or more of the inputs into this supply. The question and criteria regarding which inputs should be increased in order to increase the supply of services will be related to their relative contribution toward increased output as well as their relative costs. In order to increase any of these inputs the factors influencing their supply must be determined.

There is also a dichotomy here between the short- versus long-run supply of services and inputs. The short run is defined as that time period when it is not possible to increase all the inputs that go into the supply of dental services. Therefore any increased services in the short run must be achieved by increasing either some of the inputs and/or the time of the dentist. In the long run it is presumed that all the inputs can be increased, including the number of dentists. The time required to go from the short run to the long run depends upon how long it takes to produce dentists, the group which has the longest "gestation period" of any of the other inputs. With a given supply of dentists (the short run), the prime determinant of their supply is perhaps the additional income they could earn by working longer. The long-run supply of dentists and dental auxiliaries is the focus of much public policy concerned with increasing the supply of dental care.

The third level, below the level of supply of dental care and the number of auxiliaries and the hours worked by existing dentists and others, is the supply of training facilities for educating dentists and dental auxiliaries which determines the long-run supply of dentists. Many factors influence a person's decision to become a dentist, however; if there are insufficient educational facilities in which to provide such training (and attendance at such an institution is required in order to become a dentist) then the supply of such facilities becomes one of the most important determinants of the supply of dental manpower. Thus the third level includes the determinants of the supply of such educational facilities, and their production of graduates.

It is through these levels — the supplies of educational facilities, the supplies of dental manpower, and their determinants — that in large part determine the supply of dental services. An attempt to affect the supply of dental services must influence either the supply of training facilities and the determinants of the supply of dental manpower, or the manner in which the various inputs are combined to produce dental care — that is, what tasks can be performed by whom and whether there are changes in the level of technology. Examples of technological developments that could increase the supply of dental care would be innovations in the teaching process, which would reduce the time for producing a dentist; or improvements in equipment such as the adoption of the high speed drill, which would increase the dentist's productivity.

The Determinants of the Supply of Dental Services

Financing programs and public policy both attempt to influence each of these levels to a different degree. In order to forecast the effects of any such programs and policies we must have a better understanding of the determinants of each of these levels and how they are interrelated.

The Number of Dentists: An Overview

Much of the public policy in the dental sector has as its objective an increase in either the number of dentists or the ratio of dentists to the population. Although this emphasis on the number of dentists and on its relation to the population is incorrectly placed (as will be discussed later) it becomes important to determine the accuracy of data on the number of dentists, the factors that are likely to affect its size, and the potential availability of care from a given number of dentists.

The following sections therefore will discuss the sources of data on dentists (and discrepancies in those sources), possible biases to the total number of dentists resulting from inadequate information on foreign trained dentists and the possible effect on availability of care as a result of the increasing number of dental specialists.

Sources of Data on the Number of Dentists

There are approximately 120,000 dentists in the United States or, in terms of population per dentist, 1,685 persons per dentist (1,685:1). The number of active dentists are estimated to be approximately 104,000 or a population-dentist ratio of 1,967:1.[4]

There are two main sources for data on the number of dentists in the U.S.: the American Dental Association (ADA) and the Division of Dental Health, Department of Health, Education, and Welfare (HEW). Historically, the figures published by the Division of Dental Health were based on data collected by the ADA (as published annually in *Distribution of Dentists in the United States by State, Region, District, and County*). However, for several years, figures for total dentists published by HEW have not been in agreement with figures published by the ADA. Further, HEW publishes data on active dentists as well as on total number of dentists; the ADA only publishes data on total dentists and total nonfederal dentists. This difference between the ADA and HEW series has been more noticeable in recent years. The reasons for the divergence between these two series are as follows. The ADA publishes data annually on total dentists, total nonfederal dentists, and dental graduates in that year in their above-mentioned publication. These data are obtained via a yearly postcard survey of dentists (both ADA and nonADA members) on their status and location (conducted by the ADA's Bureau of Membership and Records). The response rate to this survey is believed, by the ADA, to be sufficiently high to place a high degree of accuracy in the results.

The original intention of the Division of Dental Health was to publish a "total dentists" figure which is calculated by subtracting the ADA's figure for "graduates" from the ADA's total for dentists in the particular year. A check of the year-by-year figures issued by HEW (in various publications) shows that in some years the HEW figures accurately match this calculation, while for other years (particularly the more recent ones) the HEW figures do not match those obtained by making the above calculation on the ADA's figures.

First, in several years HEW was required to estimate the supply of dentists prior to publication of the ADA's data. When these estimates failed to agree with the eventual ADA published figures, HEW did not change its already published figures. Also for two years (1966 and 1967) *Distribution of Dentists* was not published, thus HEW had to rely solely on its own estimates for those years.

Second, there is a difference of opinion regarding the accuracy of the ADA's published data on total dentists because it is based upon a voluntary response by the dentists to the postcard survey. Thus estimates of the stock of dentists have not been reconciled when the ADA has published its data based on its survey.

In the future, HEW hopes to publish its own complete series of dentist supply by developing its own registry of dentists in the U.S. and by revising its previous estimates of this supply.

The Division of Dental Health also publishes yearly estimates of "active" and "active nonfederal" dentists. These estimates are derived in the following fashion: using the 1950 *Census of Population,* which contained data on occupations by age, and the 1952 Dental Association register, the number of active dentists as a percentage of total dentists for each age was calculated. These percentages have then been applied annually to the data on total dentists to obtain figures for active dentists. Because the 1950 Census and 1952 ADA register were the last publications to contain accurate data of the type needed to calculate these age-group percentages, these same percentages have been used in every year since then to estimate the number of active dentists. The Division of Dental Health hopes to revise these percentages in the near future.

Data on total dentists as presented by the ADA and HEW are shown in Table 3-2. Until a data series on the number of dentists (to include both total and active dentists) is developed that is considered highly accurate by all concerned, projections of population-dentist ratios and of the available supply of dentists in some future year should be viewed with some degree of caution.

Foreign Trained Dentists

Additions to the stock of dentists may result from the in-migration of foreign trained dentists. Currently state licensing boards do not allow foreign trained dentists to practice in the United States unless they undergo additional training. This requirement applies to all foreign trained dentists except Canadian dentists. Except for five state licensing boards, Canadian dentists are permitted to

Table 3-2. Data on Population and Supply of Dentists and Population:Dentist Ratios for Selected Years, Sources and Categories

Year	Pop[2]	ADA — "Distribution of Dentists"[1]				HEW			
		Total	Total Ratio	Total Nonfederal	Total Nonfederal Ratio	Total	Total Ratio	Active	Active Ratio
1955	165,069,000	97,529	1,693:1	90,239	1,829:1	95,052[4]	1,737:1	83,509[4]	1,977:1
1958	174,149,000	101,623	1,714:1	94,649	1,840:1	98,540[5]	1,767:1	87,032[3]	2,001:1
1960	179,975,000	105,140	1,712:1	98,491	1,827:1	101,947[4]	1,765:1	89,215[4]	2,017:1
1961	182,973,000	106,554[3]	1,717:1	99,490[3]	1,839:1	103,148[3]	1,774:1	90,060[3]	2,032:1
1963	188,438,000	109,382	1,723:1	101,488	1,857:1	105,549[6]	1,785:1	91,750[3]	2,054:1
1965	193,460,000	112,455	1,720:1	104,824	1,846:1	109,320[4]	1,770:1	93,442[4]	2,070:1
1968	199,312,000	116,964	1,704:1	109,205	1,825:1	113,636[4]	1,754:1	100,010[4]	1,993:1
1970	203,736,000	120,916	1,685:1	112,879	1,805:1	118,200[4]	1,724:1	103,600[4]	1,967:1

1. American Dental Association, *Distribution of Dentists in the United States by State, Region, District, and County,* various editions.

2. *Source: Statistical Abstract of the U.S.* Figures are for "total resident population."

3. Denotes interpolation.

4. U.S. Department of Health, Education, and Welfare, Public Health Service, National Institutes of Health, Bureau of Health Manpower Education, *Manpower Supply and Educational Statistics.* PHS Publication No. 263—Sec. 20. Updated to March 3, 1971.

5. Stewart, W.A., and Pennel, Maryland Y., "Health Manpower, 1930-75," *Public Health Reports,* Vol. 75, No. 3, March 1960.

6. U.S. Department of Health, Education, and Welfare, Public Health Service, *Health Manpower Source Book: Manpower in the 1960's,* PHS Publication No. 263—Sec. 18, 1964.

practice in the states with only minimal further requirements, such as an examination.

From 1960 to 1970, a total of 2,462 foreign dentists entered the United States; 373 immigrating in 1970.[5] There is no way of determining either how many of these were Canadian dentists and thus able to enter practice after passing only a few requirements (such as an exam), or how many of the nonCanadian dentists successfully completed the substantial additional training in American schools required of them, passed the licensing exam, and then entered into practice. Again, for purposes of making projections of the likely dentist supply, it would be useful to have additional data on the increments to the total number of dentists as a result of in-migration.

The Increase in Dental Specialists

Estimates of the number of dentists and the likely availability of dental care from a given number of dentists should also take into consideration the increasing percent of dentists becoming specialists. Table 3-3 shows the increase in percent of dentists who are specialists and the relative increase in each of the specialities. Whereas in 1955 3.1 percent of dentists were specialist, in 1969 it increased to 8.5 percent. Since a specialist is not permitted to provide dental care other than in his specialty, an increase in the number of specialists might decrease the available supply of dental care if specialists were to have excess capacity.[6]

The Dentist as a Firm

The predominant form of dental practice is the solo practitioner. More than 75 percent of dentists are in a nonsalaried solo practice; less than 5 percent of dentists are organized in a group practice. Further, more than 85 percent of the practicing dentists are general practitioners.[7] The dentists in private practice may thus be viewed as the proprietor of a small competitive firm. In this role he must purchase inputs, both labor and nonlabor, and by a process of coordination and combination of these inputs, including his own time, the firm "produces" or supplies the output: dental care services. The major inputs into this production process are the dentist's time, the time of any auxiliary personnel, office expenses, equipment, and dental supplies. In those situations where the dentist is salaried the analogy to a small firm will still be appropriate, except that the function of coordination and responsibility may lie with someone else. Dental care (the output of this firm) and the productivity of the dentist are influenced by his use of these labor and nonlabor inputs. The cost of this output is affected by the cost of securing and utilizing the services of auxiliary factors as well as the cost of his office and dental supplies. Furthermore, his ability to supply output, given these inputs, will also depend upon technology and advances in technology that affect his equipment, e.g., high speed cutting drills.

If the dentist, as a firm, wanted to expand his output of dental services, he could do so in a number of ways; he could hire more auxiliaries, hence use inputs other than his own time, or he could work longer hours himself, or he could select a combination of these approaches. If there is an increase in demand for dental care, the dentist, assuming he is interested in increasing his income, will increase his output of dental services by one of the above approaches. There will thus be an increased demand for inputs (derived from the demand for dental care) and if the dentist must pay increased wages for auxiliaries or higher prices for other inputs, then his ability to increase his output of services will be limited unless the price of a visit also rises.

Similarly, if the dentist is already working the number of hours a week with which he is satisfied, the only way in which he may be induced to work more hours and increase his output would be if the price of a visit were increased, which is comparable to an increase in his wage per hour. However, at a certain point of higher prices for his additional time, and increased income, he may decide that he would prefer additional leisure to working longer hours. Beyond this point, as prices continue to rise the dentist might actually work fewer hours per week than previously. He is able to receive the same — probably higher — income with higher prices for a visit by working fewer hours than he did previously. There is some evidence (which will be presented later) that this has in fact been happening. With a given supply of dentists, therefore, increased output can continue only from increased productivity of the dentist rather than from just increased hours worked by the dentist.

Increased productivity can result from several possible sources: greater use of auxiliaries, a change in technology, or a change in the organization of the practice — possible changes in how inputs are used, for what tasks, the ability to achieve economies of scale, a change in organizational efficiency, and so forth.

To summarize the determinants of the supply of dental care, we would say that dental care can be produced with varying quantities of inputs, one of which is the dentist's own time, and that the productivity of the dentist will be affected both by the way in which these inputs are used and how many of each are used. Also affecting his productivity will be the state of technology. The cost of producing dental care is thus related to the costs of these inputs and the quantity of each used. With higher prices for dental care, the dentist is able to pay higher prices for inputs used in its production. Thus with higher prices a greater amount of care can be supplied through hiring additional inputs; it is for this reason that the relationship between quantity supplied and the price of dental care is positive, as will be shown later.

Dental Productivity — Some Empirical Evidence

The supply of dental services can be increased through either increases in the number of dentists, increases in their use of inputs, or some combination of the

Table 3-3. Number of Dental Specialists in the U.S. by Type of Specialist and as a Percent of Total Dentists, 1955-1969

Year	Total Dentists[1]	Total Specialists[2]	Endodontist[2]	Oral Pathologist[2]	Oral Surgeon[2]	Orthodontist[2]	Pedodontist[2]	Periodontist[2]	Prosthodontist[2]	Public Health Dentist[2]	Total Specialists as Percent of Total DDS
1969	118,975	10,060	478	97	2,383	4,216	1,129	951	704	102	8.46
1968	116,964	9,705	439	89	2,262	4,128	1,106	929	654	98	8.30
1965	112,455	6,462	—[3]	52	1,636	3,437	568	376	336	57	5.75
1960	105,140	4,170	—[3]	42	1,183	2,097	229	307	278	34	3.97
1955	97,529	3,034	—[3]	24	884	1,521	148	245	225	27	3.11

1. *Source:* American Dental Association, *Distribution of Dentists in the United States by State, Region, District, and County*, 1956, 1961, 1966, 1969, and 1970 issues.

2. *Source:* ADA, *Facts about States for the Dentist Seeking a Location*, 1956, 1961, 1966, 1969, and 1970 issues. All figures include dental specialists in Federal dental services.

3. The endodontists were not recognized as dental specialists in 1955 or 1960, and data are not available for 1965.

Table 3-4. Percent Changes in Dental Inputs and Outputs

	Total Patient Visits[1]		Number of Active Dentists[1]		Patient Visits per Dentist[1]		Number of Auxiliaries[1]		Auxiliaries per Dentist[1]	
	Since 1950	Since 1955	Since 1950	Since 1955	Since 1950	Since 1955	Since 1950	Since 1955	Since 1950	Since 1955
1970	82.1	48.6	33.0	24.1	36.9	19.8	79.3	47.8	34.6	18.6
1967	76.5	44.0	26.7	18.2	39.4	21.9	66.9	37.6	31.7	16.1
1964	52.6	24.5	18.9	10.9	28.4	12.3	55.4	28.1	30.8	15.3
1961	38.5	13.0	15.6	7.8	19.8	4.8	45.8	20.2	26.0	11.0
1958	34.1	9.5	11.6	4.1	20.2	5.1	34.1	10.5	20.2	5.9
1955	22.6	—	7.2	—	14.3	—	21.3	—	13.5	—
1952	—[2]	—	2.9	—	—[2]	—	8.5	—	5.8	—

1. Source for all data used to calculate percent changes: Table 3-5.   2. Data necessary to make computation unavailable.

two. For example, one approach toward increasing the supply of dental services is to increase the number of dentists, with most of the services being provided by a dentist functioning as a solo proprietor. Alternatively, an increase in output could be achieved by increasing the use of inputs, other than the number of dentists. Additional possibilities can be handled within this framework, of increasing the number of dentists or the amount of other inputs in order to achieve an increase in dental output.

In order to forecast the likely supply of dental services in some future period, it is necessary not only to be able to estimate the consequences of having fewer or more dentists but also the likely productivity of the available number of dentists. Forecasts of dental supply that ignore the effect of changes in dental productivity are likely to be inaccurate. The data indicate that over the past 20 years, increased output of dental services has resulted not so much from increases in the number of dentists but rather from their increasing productivity. This finding has two important implications, which will be discussed below: first, that increases in output can be achieved more cheaply by increasing the dentist's productivity, and second, that forecasts (hence policies) of supply of dental care using dentist-population ratios are apt to be seriously in error. The following discussion is an attempt to measure the past changes in dental productivity. Three separate measures of output are used: dental visits, consumer expenditures on dental care, and gross incomes of dentists.

Visits as a Measure of Dental Output

Table 3-4 shows the percent increase on dental output (in terms of dental visits) over time and the labor inputs, dental and auxiliary personnel, used in producing such care. The percent increase in number of dentists, from 1950 to 1970 has been 33.0 percent, while the percent increase in dental output over that time has been 82.1 percent. Since the average annual hours worked by dentists has not changed much over that time period, the increased output has been a result of increases in other inputs (as well as technology) that have changed dentists' productivity.[8]

When the data are examined in terms of annual percent increases in dental productivity we find that during 1950-1970 output increased by 1.6 percent per year. Although the earlier data are relatively less reliable (as described in the notes to Table 3-5) it appears that the increase in dental productivity has been increasing at a slightly decreasing rate. (The annual rate of increase from 1961-1970 was 1.5 percent.) The large increase in number of auxiliaries since 1950 (79.3 percent) and the consequent increase in auxiliaries per dentist (from 1.04 auxiliaries per dentist in 1950 to 1.40 in 1970) undoubtedly contributed significantly to the increase in dental output over this period. In fact the annual percentage increase in number of auxiliaries per dentist appears to be very similar to the annual percentage increase in dental productivity.

Table 3-5. Annual Percent Increase in Dental Inputs and Outputs, 1950-1970

Year	Total Patient Visits	Number of Active Dentists[1]	Patient Visits per Dentist[2]	Number of Auxiliaries[3]	Auxiliaries per Dentist	Annual Percent Increase in Visits per D.D.S.		Annual Percent Increase in Auxiliaries per D.D.S.	
						Since 1950	Since 1955	Since 1950	Since 1955
1970	369,334,000	103,600	3,565	145,200	1.40	1.6	1.2	1.5	1.1
1967	358,073,430	98,670	3,629	135,180	1.37	2.0	1.7	1.6	1.3
1964	309,551,771	92,597	3,343	125,900	1.36	1.8	1.3	1.9	1.6
1961	280,897,140	90,060	3,119	118,100	1.31	1.7	0.8	2.1	1.7
1958	272,100,290	86,933	3,130	108,600	1.25	2.3	1.7	2.3	1.9
1955	248,606,293	83,509	2,977	98,250	1.18	2.7	—	2.6	—
1952	—[4]	80,144	—[4]	87,900	1.10	—[4]	—	2.8	—
1950	202,851,600	77,900	2,604[5]	81,000	1.04	—	—	—	—

1. *Source:* U.S. Department of Health, Education, and Welfare, Public Health Service, National Institutes of Health, Bureau of Health Manpower Education, Division of Dental Health, Manpower Studies Branch, *Health Manpower Source Book: Section 20, Manpower Supply and Educational Statistics*, updated as of March, 1971. PHS Publication No. 263-20 pp. 25, 38. This contains data for years 1950, 1955, 1960, 1965-1970. Years 1952, 1958, 1961, 1964 in this table are interpolations on this data.

2. *Source:* American Dental Association, *Survey of Dental Practice*, 1950, 1956, 1959, 1962, 1965, 1968, 1971.

3. *Source:* Based on correspondence with Ruth Bothwell, Division of Dental Health, Public Health Service, Department of Health, Education, and Welfare. Data for years 1950 1960, 1965, 1970; years 1952, 1958, 1961, 1964, 1967 in the table are interpolations of this data. It should be noted that the data presented on auxiliaries differ from estimates of the number of auxiliaries published in the ADA's *Survey of Dental Practice*. The ADA data are: 1971: 154,500 full-time and 50,800 part-time auxiliaries; 1968: 136,400 and 37,800; 1965: 116,300 and 28,000; 1962: 91,100 and 30,900; 1958: 77,500 and 36,700; 1955: 82,500 full-time, no estimate for part-time; 1952: 64,500; 1950: 61,200. Also, in early years the data excluded secretaries.

4. Data not available.

5. This figure is relatively unreliable because it was calculated as the product of "mean weeks worked per year" times "mean patient visits in sample week." Other figures in this column are actual averages, as found in *Survey of Dental Practice.*

Admittedly such aggregate time series data does not make it possible to hold constant other factors which have changed over this period, such as the type of dental service being provided, the age of the dentist, the average number of hours worked (which appears to have fallen sharply since the mid-1960s) and technological changes. The main contribution to increased dental productivity, based on these time series data, appear to have been the increased use of auxiliaries. If more data of a less aggregate nature were available it might indicate that the effect of auxiliaries was even greater than shown since the number of dental hours worked decreased and the composition of the mix of dental treatments changed; meaning that an average visit today presumably requires more time than the average visit 10 or 20 years ago. This change in the composition of the mix of dental visits is indicated by the change in weights given to the data on fees collected by the ADA in constructing their "Composite Fee"[9]

In order to have a clearer look at the increase in dental productivity that is possible as a result of increased use of auxiliary personnel, a cross sectional analysis of such data was examined. Tables 3-6 and 3-7 show the number of auxiliary persons per dentist, and dental output measured in terms of numbers of visits per dentist. This same data is also shown for different time periods.

Table 3-6. Average Annual Patient Visits per Dentist by Number of Auxiliary Personnel Employed

Year[1]	Auxiliaries Employed (Full-time Personnel Only)[6]				
	0	1	2	3	4 or more
1958[3]	2272	3014	3174	3929	—[2]
1961[4]	2003	2968	3706	4790	—[2]
1964[5]	2355	3015	3946	4409	6170

1. Data incomplete, unavailable, or unreliable for 1950, 1953, 1956, and 1968, *Surveys of Dental Practice.*

2. Too few Survey replies for reliable statistics.

3. *Source:* American Dental Association, *The 1959 Survey of Dental Practice,* p. 47.

4. *Source:* American Dental Association, *The 1962 Survey of Dental Practice,* p. 45.

5. *Source:* American Dental Association, *The 1965 Survey of Dental Practice,* p. 35.

6. Auxiliaries include dental technicians, dental hygienists, dental assistants, and secretaries/receptionists.

The data are consistent in that they show that a given dentist can achieve significant increases in his output with the use of auxiliary personnel. Further, it is certainly in the dentist's economic interest to use such personnel, since the contribution to his income from additional auxiliaries is positive (as will be discussed in a later section). Depending upon the number of auxiliaries added, the percent increase in output with each auxiliary varies between 20 and 40 percent. Also, Table 3-8 shows that proportionately more dentists have been

Table 3-7. Mean Increase in Average Annual Patient Visits per Dentist per Additional Auxiliary Employed[1]

	0	1	2	3	4 or more[4]
Mean Patient Visits per Dentist[2]	2210	2999	3609	4376	6170
Increase in Patient Visits from Addition of Auxiliary	–	789	610	767	1794
Percentage Increase in Patient Visits[3]	–	35.7	20.4	21.3	41.0

1. "Auxiliary Personnel" include dental technicians, dental hygienists, dental assistants, and secretary-receptionists.

2. Based on data from American Dental Association, *Survey of Dental Practice,* 1959, 1962, 1965. Mean is for years 1955, 1961, and 1964. See Table 3-6.

3. Percentage Increase = $\dfrac{\text{Increase}}{\text{Previous Value}}$

4. Too few replies in 1959 and 1962 *Surveys* for reliable statistics, therefore, "Mean" is simply figure for 1964 and increase in visits from 3 to 4 auxiliaries are based only on 1964 figure.

increasing their use of such auxiliaries over time. The data appear, therefore, to substantiate the hypothesis that large increases in dental output over time have resulted from increased use of auxiliaries. The contribution to increased output by other inputs, such as increased capital and technological changes, might be seen when we examine the increase in number of patient visits per dentist with two and three auxiliaries over time as shown in Table 3-6. The average number of dental hours worked was similar for both 1961 and 1964; the 1958 average dental hours worked were greater than the later years, therefore it should be excluded from the comparison. This increase in output per dentist between 1961 and 1964, which is in the neighborhood of several hundred visits per year per dentist, might be considered the additional output that is caused by increases in technology and capital. (The tentative nature of these conclusions should be kept in mind because of the small number of years involved.)

An Index of Real Output Based on Deflated Consumer Expenditures

Another method used to estimate the change in output per dentist is to deflate consumer expenditures for dental care by the dental care price index. Weiss[10] constructed an index of real output of dental services for 1935-1963 and estimated the average annual productivity increase by all dentists (which consisted of the adjusted for price changes expenditure data on a per dentist

Table 3-8. Percent Distribution of Dentists by Number of Full-time Auxiliary Personnel Employed[1]

Year	Full-time Auxiliaries Employed[2]				
	0	1	2	3	4 or more
1950[3]	34.4	54.3	8.5	1.9	0.9
1952[4]	29.2	50.2	9.9	1.9	8.8
1955[5]	24.3	51.3	13.3	3.1	8.0
1958[6]	–	–	–	–	–
1961[7]	21.9	46.6	10.0	21.5	
1964[8]	13.6	40.6	10.8	1.5	33.5
1967[9]	10.2	34.3	15.0	1.9	39.6
1970[10]	10.1	25.7	11.2	6.3	45.3

1. Figures may not add to 100 percent for any particular year due to omission of dentists classified as employing "part-time" auxiliary personnel.

2. "Auxiliary personnel" include dental technicians, dental hygienists, dental assistants, and secretary-receptionists.

3. *Source:* American Dental Association, *Survey of the Dental Profession, 1950,* p. 15.

4. *Source:* ADA, *The 1953 Survey of Dental Practice,* p. 26.

5. *Source:* ADA, *The 1956 Survey of Dental Practice,* p. 21.

6. Data not available in *The 1959 Survey of Dental Practice.*

7. *Source:* ADA, *The 1962 Survey of Dental Practice,* p. 28.

8. *Source:* ADA, *The 1965 Survey of Dental Practice,* p. 22.

9. *Source:* ADA, *The 1968 Survey of Dental Practice,* p. 20.

10. *Source:* ADA, "The 1971 Survey of Dental Practice V. Auxiliary Personnel," *JADA,* June, 1972, p. 1375. This data comes from Table 28, and is consistent with the data for the earlier years. However, in Table 27 of page 1375, the ADA for the first time published a percent distribution of dentists by member of auxiliary personnel employed for all types and combinations of auxiliaries. These figures are: "0" full-time auxiliaries, 16.8 percent; "1" full-time auxiliary, 33.7 percent; "2" full-time auxiliaries, 24.6 percent; "3" full-time auxiliaries, 11.8 percent; "4" full-time auxiliaries, 5.3 percent; "5" full-time auxiliaries, 1.6 percent; "6" full-time auxiliaries, 3.1 percent; others, 4.6 percent.

The reason for a discrepancy between these figures and those published in the tables is that except for 1950, this table was compiled by examining *Survey* tables listing percentages of dentists using various employee mixes, such as "two assistants" or "one assistant and one hygienist," and adding percentages from those categories representing use of *x* auxiliaries (e.g., both classifications mentioned above were lumped under "2 auxiliaries"). "Part-time" employees were disregarded; thus a classification in the *Survey* such as "one assistant and one part-time assistant" was listed in our table as "1 (full-time) auxiliary." Also, in the *Survey* tables, an "other" category was listed. We have placed this category under "4 or more full-time auxiliaries employed" in our table (or, in the case of 1961 where data was given for neither "3" nor "4", "others" has been lumped under "3" *and* "4"). This undoubtedly has imparted an upward bias to the data, since "others" probably represents not only those dentists utilizing 4 or more auxiliary employees, but also those dentists utilizing lesser numbers of auxiliaries whose "mixes" are not given in the *Survey* data. For example, the classification "one hygienist and one secretary or receptionist" was not given in the *Survey* tables, instead being lumped in with "others." Had this classification appeared in the *Survey* data, it would have been added to our category "2 full-time auxiliaries employed"; however, since it appears in the *Survey* data only as a part of "others," this classification has been incorporated into our category "4 or more full-time auxiliaries employed."

basis) for the period 1950-1963 to be 2.83 percent and for the period 1955-1961 to be 2.10 percent. We have extended the calculations of real expenditures for dental care to 1970, and, by dividing real dental expenditures by the number of active dentists, we have calculated a measure of real output per dentist and the annual percentage increase in real output per dentist for the periods 1950, 1960, and 1970. These data are shown in Table 3-9.

Table 3-9. An Index of Real Output Using Deflated Expenditures for Dental Care 1950, 1960, and 1970

Year	Adjusted Consumer Expenditures[1]	Expenditures per D.D.S.	Percent Increase in Expenditures per D.D.S. Since 1950	Annual Percent Increase in Expenditures per D.D.S. Since 1950
1970	$2,915,000,000	$28,137	85.8	3.1
1960	$1,917,000,000	$21,487	41.9	3.6
1950	$1,180,000,000	$15,148	–	–

1. Adjusted by Dental Care Price Index, with 1957-1959 = 100.

Annual increases in dental productivity appear to be much greater when expenditure data are used than when visits are used as the measure of output. From 1950 to 1960, real output per dentist increased 41.9 percent using expenditures as a proxy for output and only 20.0 percent when visits were used. (The annual percentage increase in productivity from 1950-1960 was 3.6 and 1.8 respectively.) Since 1960, expenditure data continued to show larger increases in real output than output increases based on visit data. From 1950-1970 the annual percentage increase in productivity has been 3.1 based on expenditures while it has been only 1.6 percent using visit data. The increase in output per dentist from 1950-1970 was 88.5 percent and 36.9 percent using expenditures and visit data respectively.

As a possible explanation for differences in real output when expenditures as compared to visits are used as the measure of output, an examination was made of the Dental Care Price Index. If actual dental prices increased more rapidly in the period 1950-1970 than was indicated by the Dental Care Price Index (published by the Bureau of Labor Statistics), then the real increase in output as measured by BLS adjusted data would be overstated.

In collecting more recent data from the BLS for their dental price index, it was discovered that they had revised their base year, from 1957 to 1967. This revised BLS "fee" series is presented in Table 3-10, for the same years for which data on fees were available from ADA sources.

The American Dental Association collects data on mean fees for different dental treatments in its periodic *Surveys on Dental Practice.* A composite fee is then calculated by the ADA using various weights for the different fees. In order to compare the increases in fees based on data collected by the ADA in its surveys to those of the Bureau of Labor Statistics, certain revisions had to be

Table 3-10. Indices of Dental Prices, 1956-1970 (1967 = 100)[1]

Year	BLS: "Dentists' Fees"[2]	ADA: Composite (Weight 1)[4]	ADA: Composite (Weight 2)[5]	ADA: Complete Upper Denture[3]	ADA: Filling, Amalgam, 1 Surface[3]	ADA: Prophylaxis[3]	ADA: Single Extraction[3]	ADA: Acrylic Jacket Crown[3]
1970	119.4	122.59	121.45	121.51	120.10	127.16	128.82	114.56
1968	105.5	105.84	105.60	104.69	106.75	105.62	106.22	105.33
1967	100.0	100.00	100.00	100.00	100.00	100.00	100.00	100.00
1965	92.2	88.35	88.81	90.64	86.66	88.78	87.43	89.36
1962	84.7	80.37	80.87	81.99	80.07	81.47	77.97	81.33
1959	80.5	73.38	72.87	75.68	74.54	74.29	70.63	69.73
1956	74.4	66.84	66.67	67.28	70.25	66.45	62.15	66.27

1. In order to make the ADA and BLS series comparable, the ADA data were interpolated so that 1967 was the base year.

2. *Source:* Martin Smith, U.S. Department of Labor, Bureau of Labor Statistics. The Bureau of Labor Statistics publishes a price index entitled "Dentists' Fees." This series is calculated by weighting the prices for "fillings, adult, amalgam, one surface," "extractions, adult," and "dentures, full upper" by a set of "cost weights." These weights represent the percentage of total consumer dental expenditures spent on each of weights represent the percentage of total consumer dental expenditures spent on each of these three services, respectively, excluding all other types of dental services. In other words, the three weights always sum to one, and the percent expenditures on these services these services are calculated relative to each other. No adjustment is made for the fact that, for example, expenditures for another service such as prophylaxis may increase as a percentage of total expenditures in a given period, while expenditures for fillings, extractions, and dentures decrease as a percentage of total expenditures.

These cost weights were developed from the data collected in the Consumer Expenditure Survey of 1961-1962. The weights are adjusted monthly according to price movements in the dental sector. Another Consumer Expenditure Survey is currently being conducted, thus we may soon expect a recalculation of the base weights.

Before 1964, only data on fillings and extractions were used in calculating the "Dentists' Fees" price index. Thus the series "Dentist Fees" for years before 1964 represents only the weighted prices of fillings and extractions (with the weights again summing to one).

Price indices for the three component services are also published by the BLS. The series for "Complete Upper Denture" only extends back to 1964, which was the first year in which fee data for this service was collected.

3. *Sources:* ADA, Bureau of Economic Research and Statistics, "Dental Fees in 1956, 1959, 1962, 1965, 1968," *Journal of the American Dental Association,* October, 1957; April, 1961; November, 1963; August, 1966; June, 1969; and "National Dental Fee Survey, 1970," *JADA,*

July, 1971. (Data on mean fees for each type of service.) This data for 1956-1968 was collected by the ADA via the *Survey of Dental Practice* questionnaires for those years. Data on 1 surface amalgam filling was not collected by the ADA for 1968, therefore an estimate was derived by interpolation.

4. Calculated by multiplying each fee times its weight, then summing. These weights, which were used by the ADA from 1962-1968, are: complete upper denture, 1; filling, amalgam, 1 surface, 30; prophylaxis, 10; single extraction, 20; acrylic jacket crown, 1. *Source: JADA*, June, 1972, p. 1382.

The composite fee as calculated by us is not the same as the "mean composite fee" as calculated by the American Dental Association. For some years, this is due to the fact that we have used a different weighting system than has the ADA. In some years, however, we have used the same weights as the ADA, yet still obtained a different figure for the composite fee. This is because our composite fee is calculated by multiplying each mean fee by its weight, then summing; whereas the ADA's mean composite fee is the mean of the composite fees calculated for each responding dentist who provided data on all five fees. The difference lies in the fact that the mean for each individual fee includes data from dentists who provided information on that particular fee, but not necessarily on all of the fees. Any responding dentist who provided data on less than all of the fees was not included by the ADA in computation of its mean composite fee, but was included in the computation of the means for those individual fees on which he supplied a figure. Thus, our composite fee is derived from a slightly different sample than is the ADA's mean composite fee.

5. Calculated by multiplying each fee times its weight, then summing. These weights, which are *currently* used by the ADA, are: complete upper denture, 1; filling, amalgam, 1 surface, 19; prophylaxis, 22; single extraction, 13; acrylic jacket crown, 3. *Source: JADA*, June, 1972, p. 1382. See footnote 4 for explanation of differences between composite fees as claculated by us and by the ADA.

Table 3-11. Annual Percent Increase in Expenditures per Active Dentist, Deflated by BLS and ADA Price Series[1]

Year	Consumer Expenditures for Dental Care	Real Expenditures as Deflated by BLS "Dentists' Fees" Index	Real Expenditures as Deflated by ADA "Composite Fee" Index #1	BLS: Real Expenditures per Active D.D.S.	ADA: Real Expenditures per Active D.D.S.	BLS Annual Percent Increase in Real Expenditures per Active D.D.S.	ADA Annual Percent Increase in Real Expenditures per Active D.D.S.
1970	$4,211,000,000	$3,526,800,670	$3,435,027,327	$34,042	$33,157	2.9	2.7
1960	$1,962,000,000	$2,389,768,575	$2,513,451,191	$26,786	$28,173	3.4	3.9
1950	$ 961,000,000	$1,503,912,363	$1,503,912,363	$19,306	$19,306	—	—

1. Base period is 1967.

made to the ADA data. The reasons for these revisions and the method used to make the two series comparable are explained in the footnotes to Table 3-10, which shows a comparison of dental fees between the BLS and the ADA data. As can be seen from this table, dental prices, as measured by the BLS increased from 80.5 in 1959 to 119.4 in 1970.

For the same period, dental prices (as measured by the ADA) increased from 73.3 to 122.59, thereby indicating a more rapid rise in dental fees when ADA data are used. The data on consumer expenditures for dental care were then adjusted by both the BLS (revised) fee series and the ADA fee series, as shown in Table 3-11. The annual percentage increase in real expenditures per active dentist from 1950-1970 are, however, similar when using either the BLS or ADA adjusted expenditures. For BLS adjusted data it is 2.9 percent, while for the ADA adjusted data it is 2.7 percent. Both these series of annual percentage increases in productivity are still higher than the estimates using ADA visit data, which was 1.6 percent per year for the period 1950-1970.

Thus the BLS price series, with 1957 as the base year, would appear to indicate higher annual percentage increases in dental productivity than when the expenditures data are deflated using the BLS *revised* (1967 as the base period) fee series.

It appears however that the annual percentage increases in dental productivity when using either adjusted expenditures or visit data was higher in the period 1950-1960 (3.4 percent) than it was from 1960-1970 (2.4 percent per year, using BLS adjusted series). The comparable percent increases using ADA adjusted expenditures are 3.9 percent per year from 1950-1960 and 1.6 percent per year from 1960-1970.

An Index of Production Based on Gross Incomes of Dentists

Another proxy measure of dental care output is the gross income of the dentists. If the price of dental care was similar among dentists employing different numbers of auxiliary personnel (and in their use of other inputs and technology) for a given time period, then differences in gross incomes are a result of differences in dental output. An index of production based on this method was presented in Appendix A of the *Survey of Dentistry*.

According to Table 3-12 the gross income of dentists employing no auxiliaries is used as the base for each year and is equal to 100.00. The gross income of each dentist-auxiliary combination is then divided by the gross income of dentists with no auxiliaries and this percentage is then the index for that particular dentist-auxiliary combination. Thus the difference in indices within each year is the percentage increase in productivity attributed to increased use of auxiliaries. For example, in 1964, dentists employing one auxiliary were on the average about 71 percent more productive than were dentists with no employees; dentists employing two auxiliaries were on the average about 152 percent more productive than were dentists with no employees, and so on.

Table 3-12. Index of Production by Number of Auxiliaries Employed by Gross Income of Dentists

Number of Auxiliaries Employed	1952	1955	1958	1961	1964	1967	1970
0	100.00	100.00	100.00	100.00	100.00	100.00	100.00
1	174.74	174.12	163.22	180.67	170.84	155.73	133.16
2	257.46	248.66	228.60	268.97	252.33	224.52	191.81
3	342.87	318.91	301.45	344.18	339.40	280.71	261.30
4	501.37	379.66	416.26	461.14	450.20	342.07	318.44

Source: ADA, *Survey of Dental Practice*, 1953, 1956, 1959, 1962, 1965, 1968, 1971.

For each of the years presented the data are consistent in that they show that a given dentist can achieve significant increases in his output with the use of auxiliary personnel. Depending upon the number of auxiliaries added, the percentage increase in output with each additional auxiliary will vary, and in the more recent years appears to decline for each dental-auxiliary combination.

Another approach (using dentists' gross income) that attempted to measure the change in dentists' productivity over time was that used by Maurizi.[11] Using gross dental income per hour, adjusted for increases in dental fees, Maurizi arrived at an annual increase in dental productivity of 2.2 percent between 1955 and 1961, thus placing him in accord with the findings of Weiss of 2.1 percent for the same period using real expenditures for dental care.

Extending Maurizi's approach for a longer period of time and using more recent data the following results were derived, as shown in Table 3-13. (The years for which data are presented are from the ADA's *Surveys of Dental Practice.*) As seen in the table, the annual percentage increase in gross income per hour has been increasing since 1955. For example, as of 1970, gross income per hour has increased 7.2 percent annually since 1955. When this estimate is adjusted by the increase in dental fees, which has also been rising annually, the real annual increase in productivity has been 3.1 percent since 1955. Since the estimates of the annual percentage increase in dental productivity presented earlier used 1950 as the base year, this estimate of 3.1 percent since 1955 appears to be similar to the other estimates based upon adjusted expenditures.

Contribution to Increased Productivity
from Technological Change

There are several difficulties in separating out the increases in dentist productivity attributable to various factors other than increased use of auxiliaries. If one were to compare the differences in number of visits over time for each combination of dentists and auxiliaries, it would be necessary to hold constant differences in hours worked by the dentists, which have changed over time. When productivity is measured by either gross income of the dentist or in terms of real expenditures for dental care, then in addition to variations in hours worked there is a problem of possibly different dental fees by different dentist-auxiliary combinations. In other words, prices charged may vary according to who performs the service. Thus it becomes difficult to estimate the relative contribution of the various components that have led to increased dental productivity.

There have, however, been several attempts to estimate the effects of factors other than increased use of auxiliaries on dental productivity. One such study estimated the time saved, hence additional caries filled and bridges placed, of using high speed cutting equipment. "The total theoretical saving of dentists'

Table 3-13. Annual Dentist Productivity Increases, Measured in Terms of Gross Income of Dentists per Hour Worked

Year	Mean Gross Income[1]	Annual Mean Hours Worked[1]	Gross Income per Hour	Composite Fee (#1)[2]	Annual Percent Change in Gross Income per Hour	Since 1955	
						Annual Percent Change in Composite Fee	Annual Percent Change in Productivity[4]
1970	$59,325	1,949.9	$30.42	$785.49	7.2	4.1	3.1
1967	$46,391	2,023.8	$22.92	$678.16	6.4	3.9	2.5
1964	$36,352	2,039.0	$17.83	$566.09	5.7	3.1	2.6
1961	$29,435	2,038.3	$14.44	$515.00	4.9	3.1	1.8
1958	$26,030	2,090.4	$12.45	$470.18	4.7	3.2	1.5
1955	$22,093	2,039.0	$10.84	$428.27	—	—	—
1952	$18,797	2,013.5	$ 9.34	—[3]	—	—	—

1. *Source:* American Dental Association, *Survey of Dental Practice,* 1953, 1956, 1959, 1962, 1965, 1968, 1971.

2. *Source:* ADA, Bureau of Economic Research and Statistics, "Dental Fees in 1956, 1959, 1962, 1965, 1968," *Journal of the American Dental Association,* October, 1957; April, 1961; November, 1963; August, 1966; June, 1969; and "National Dental Fee Survey, 1970," *JADA,* July, 1971 (data on fees by type of service). The weighting schedule used was the one used by the ADA in 1962-1965. See Table 3-10, footnote 4.

3. Fee data unavailable, hence the composite fee could not be calculated.

4. Calculation: [Annual percent change in gross income per hour since 1955] − [Annual percent change in composite fee since 1955].

time from the use of high speed equipment is, therefore, the equivalent of 1,741 dentists (over the period 1950-1975)."[12] Assuming (among other things) that the number of dentists in 1975 were to be approximately 115,000, then this savings would represent a 1.5 percent average annual increase in dental productivity.

Maurizi also attempted to measure the annual percent increase in dental productivity attributable to technical change over time.[13] He compared the change in dentist time input required to perform various types of services between 1943-1950 and between 1943-1958 (the only years for which any of the necessary data were available). The result of his calculations was that technical change increased output by approximately 1 percent per year over the period 1943-1958, while for the period 1943-1950 the average annual increase was greater — approximately 1.3 percent per year. Using some of the earlier data, Maurizi adjusted the dentist time input by age of dentists and derived a second estimate of technical change equal to .84 percent per year.

Summary of Empirical Evidence on Dental Productivity

In summary, increases in dental productivity over the last twenty years have contributed significantly to the increase in the output of dental services. When dental services are measured in terms of patient visits, the annual percentage increase in dental productivity has been 1.6 percent. If adjusted consumer expenditures are used, then the annual increase in productivity has been 3.1 percent. The last measure used as a proxy for dental services was gross incomes of dentists. When adjusted by price increases, gross incomes of dentists have risen 3.1 percent per year from 1955-1970.

It appears that the annual percentage increase in dental productivity in the last several years has not been as large as it was previously. A possible explanation for this observation is the decrease in dental hours worked and the change in the composition of a patient visit. Fewer visits, with a longer average time per visit, will suggest a decrease in productivity if the outcome measure were not adjusted for differences in time. A change in what constitutes a visit may also explain the differences in annual productivity increases when visit data are used comapred to when dental services are measured by expenditures or gross incomes. The latter measures would be more likely to incorporate the change in visits, hence might be a more accurate estimate of the annual percentage change in dental productivity.

The findings with respect to the influence of technical change on dental productivity based on the study by Maurizi, the estimates in the 1961 *Survey of Dentistry*, and the analysis of differences in patient visits for different dental-auxiliary combinations between 1961 and 1964, are for the most part of a highly tentative nature, but suggest an annual increase in dental productivity of approximately 1 percent per year. The remaining annual increase in dental productivity (1-2 percent) would be attributable to factors affecting the scale of the dentist's practice such as additional auxiliary personnel, and chairs.

There are additional factors that could result in economies as size of office practice is increased, namely, if dentists were to organize in some form of group practice. There might be savings from sharing of personnel as well as in financial (billing, accounting) and capital aspects of the practice.[14] Data from each of the ADA's *Survey of Dental Practice* indicate that net incomes of dentists that share the costs of offices or assistants are higher than those that do not.

We might infer therefore that increased use of auxiliaries per dentist and the sharing of other fixed resources will result in economies as size of practice is increased. However, the "optimal" size of practice (most economically efficient) is probably on a relatively small scale because of current restrictive practices with regard to the delegation of certain tasks. Also, a dentist's incentive to work longer decreases if he is only one of a large number of dentists sharing the revenue from the practice than if his increased productivity directly increases income for him.[15]

Nevertheless it would be worthwhile to conduct additional studies of economies of scale in dental practices, allowing for differences in the product mix between different sized settings. Studies of economies of scale of physician's practice which would have some similarity to that of the dentist, are either inconclusive or show only small economies from increasing the size of the practice.[16]

Factors Influencing the Use of Auxiliary Personnel

Once the dentist begins to add auxiliaries, the nature of his job changes, more of his time is spent at the chair, his hours in the laboratory decrease, as do his free hours in the office.[17] In addition to delegating some of his tasks to auxiliaries he will also use outside commercial laboratories instead of doing such tasks himself. This tendency to substitute lesser skilled personnel in doing tasks, and to purchase services rather than produce them himself, all tend to increase his productivity, thereby increasing his output and hence his income. The data clearly support what many people have been saying for years — that it is possible and profitable for dentists to increase their output in a number of ways, foremost among them being an increase in the number of auxiliaries they employ.

Why, then, don't dentists employ more auxiliaries? Part of the reason is a lack of knowledge about how to use such persons; and, those who were trained to use auxiliaries may have gotten out of the habit after being in a new practice by themselves for a number of years. However, we believe the majority of dentists understand the implications of auxiliaries and techniques to increase their productivity. The reason that auxiliaries are not used to their fullest is because of insufficient demand. A dentist in private practice presumably would prefer to work a minimum number of hours a week in order to earn a certain income. If, at current dental prices, there is insufficient demand for his services it will be less costly for him to perform all the tasks himself, rather than hire auxiliaries. If, however, the demand for his services begins to increase, then he will hire an assistant and additional personnel as necessary, if their contribution to revenue is greater than the additional expense of employing them.

This hypothesis appears to be accurate as shown in the data on "busyness" of the dentist and the mean number of days spent waiting for an appointment by patients. Based on ADA *Surveys of Dental Practice,* the use of personnel by dentists has increased over time along with patient waiting times and the "busyness" of the dentist, while the number of dentists indicating that they would like to work more hours has been decreasing. These measures suggest that demand has been increasing at all levels and that this is an important reason for the increased use of auxiliaries over time.

If this is what has been occuring, then we might hypothesize that as demand for dental care continues to increase (as discussed in Chapter 2) we would then expect to observe an increase in the demand for auxiliaries and the greater employment of them. With continued increases in the demand for dental care, the number of auxiliaries to be employed per dentist would be related to several factors, among which would be the cost of employing them, the price of dental care, and how much and what type of care the auxiliary can provide. Related to this latter aspect are the types of restrictions that are placed on auxiliaries regarding the types of care that they can provide.

Currently, strong restrictions exist with regard to auxiliary functions. As long as the demand facing each dentist is not sufficiently large so that within the restrictions provided by current regulations he can delegate some tasks and still provide the remainder of those services himself, he can still increase his productivity by increasing his use of auxiliary personnel. But once the demand increases beyond the point which the dentist having several auxiliaries can handle, it would be difficult, according to the regulations, to increase his output much further with additional auxiliaries, unless he can delegate more tasks to them than are currently permitted under vitually all state regulations.

This analysis suggests that as demand for dental care increases we will continue to observe increased use of auxiliaries, hence increased output and increased dental productivity, primarily from those dentists who are currently low in their use of auxiliaries. If current restrictions on dental tasks persist, however, prospects for continued increases in productivity will be diminished after a certain level of demand has occurred and a certain size of practice has been achieved. We would therefore expect that as demand for dental care continues to increase there would be support from the dental profession for a lessening of the restrictions currently placed on auxiliaries. As long as the auxiliary must work under the control of the dentist, then such a policy would increase the dentist's productivity, hence his income.

Revised Estimates of Dental Supply

Estimates of impending shortages of dental supply have traditionally used dental population ratios as proxies for the available supply. The implicit assumption underlying such an approach is that increases in supply must be achieved in terms of a fixed ratio of dentists to population. However, if increases in supply can be achieved by increasing the dentist's productivity, as has been discussed above, then a smaller dentist-population ratio will be required. If the supply increase is achieved by increases in the number of dentists, then this is not only a more costly approach but also takes longer to achieve, since the training time for producing a dentist is much longer than for an auxiliary. Since large increases in productivity are possible with increased use of auxiliaries, estimates of future requirements for dentists in order to meet increased demands for dental services should be revised. Such a revised estimate would include the increase in available supply reflecting the increased number of auxiliaries per dentist.

Table 3-14 shows the increase in patient visits per year which could be realized if each dentist had either three or four auxiliary employees (for those dentists using fewer than that number). The table indicates the percent of "potential" capacity at which the dental services industry was operating during different years. The construction of this table is based upon an earlier table showing the percent of dentists using different number of auxiliaries at different periods of time. It is apparent that the trend over time is toward greater utilization of auxiliaries by dentists. The percentage of dentists employing no full-time auxiliary personnel decreased from 34.4 percent in 1950 to 10.1 percent in 1970; the percentage of dentists employing only one full-time auxiliary also decreased between 1950 and 1970, from 54.3 percent to 25.7 percent. In this same period the percentage of dentists employing two full-time auxiliaries increased from 8.5 percent to 11.2 percent. Because of the uncertain effect of the "others" category listed under "3" and "4" full-time auxiliary employees, inferences drawn from this end of the table would probably be meaningless. However, we would expect that the percentages of dentists employing both three and four full-time auxiliaries has also increased from 1950 to 1970.

The construction of this table assumes that each dentist would have the necessary office space and equipment to utilize fully his additional full-time auxiliary personnel. It further assumes that all "auxiliaries" and "auxiliary mixes" are equally productive, whereas in fact a combination of, for example, one technician, one assistant, and one secretary might differ in productivity from a combination of two assistants and one secretary. In other words, the table indicates the increase in provision of dental services which could be realized by supplying each dentist with additional "capital" and "labor," regardless of possible constraints on the supply of dentists.

For example in 1958, dentists provided only 71.5 percent of the potential visits possible if each one of them had employed three full-time auxiliaries, and only 50.7 percent of the visits possible if they had each employed four full-time auxiliaries. Four full-time auxiliaries were used as a maximum since it was indicated that this was an "optimum" number of persons to be employed by each dentist.[18] Note that there has been an increase over time in both total patient visits and in percent of "potential" capacity used. This indicates that in

Table 3-14. Unused Capacity to Provide Dental Services, Based on Maximum Utilization of Full-Time Auxiliary Personnel [1, 8, 9]

Year	Total Patient Visits[2]	Total Possible Visits 3 Auxiliaries per Dentist[3]	Percent	Total Possible Visits 4 Auxiliaries per Dentist[5]	Percent Capacity[4]
1950	175,820,300[7]	340,890,400	51.6	480,643,000	36.6
1952	—[10]	350,692,640	—[10]	494,463,800	—[10]
1955	250,276,473	365,436,384	68.5	515,250,530	48.6
1958	272,134,720	380,466,944	71.5	536,444,480	50.7
1961	280,881,545	394,080,680	71.3	555,639,350	50.6
1964	309,551,771	405,204,472	76.4	571,323,490	54.2
1967	358,073,430	431,779,920	82.9	608,793,900	58.8
1970	369,334,000	453,353,600	81.5	639,212,000	57.8

1. All figures obtained or derived from data obtained from the American Dental Association, *Survey of Dental Practice,* 1950, 1953, 1956, 1962, 1965, 1968; with exception noted in footnote 9 below.

2. Calculation: mean annual patient visits per dentist in year x times active practicing dentists in year x.

3. Calculation: mean annual patient visits per dentist for 1958, 1961, 1964 (see Table 3-7) of dentists employing 3 auxiliaries times active practicing dentists in year x.

4. Calculation: $\dfrac{\text{total patient visits in year } x}{\text{total possible visits, 3 aux. per dentist, in year } x} \times 100$

5. Calculation: mean annual patient visits per dentist employing 4 auxiliaries for 1964 (see Table 3-7) times active participating dentists in year x.

6. Calculation: $\dfrac{\text{total patient visits in year } x}{\text{total possible visits, 4 aux. per dentist, in year } x} \times 100$

7. Figure derived from data in *Survey of the Dental Profession 1950,* pp. 21, 22, 24. Calculation involved determining total dentists using y chairs (percent using y chairs times active dentists in 1950, 77,900); multiplying the total dentists using each amount of chairs by the mean patients per week by number of chairs used (this is equal to mean patient visits per week by number of chairs used if it is assumed a patient will only come once in a week); these products were then summed and multiplied by 46.5 (average number of weeks worked per dentist in 1949) to get total visits in 1950.

8. "Auxiliary personnel" include dental technicians, dental hygienists, dental assistants, and secretary receptionists.

9. Data on active dentists in year x used to make calculations obtained from *Manpower Supply and Educational Statistics for Dentists and Dental Auxiliaries,* March 3, 1971, published by U.S. Department of Health, Education, and Welfare, Public Health Service, National Institutes of Health, Bureau of Manpower Education, p. 25. For years where this figure was not given in the above source (1952, 1958, 1961, 1964) straight-line interpolation was used on the given data.

10. Data on patient visits unobtainable in *The 1953 Survey of Dental Practice.*

the period 1950 to 1970 the trend was toward greater utilization of auxiliary personnel by dentists. In 1970 the percent of "potential" capacity used in the industry had risen to 81.5 percent and 57.8 percent, as compared to 51.6 and 36.6 in 1951, with three and four auxiliaries per dentist, respectively.

Since "total possible visits, 3 auxiliaries per dentist" is based on mean patient visits per year per dentist with 3 full-time auxiliaries for 1958, 1961, and 1964, and "total possible visits, 4 auxiliaries per dentist" is based on mean patient visits per year per dentist with 4 full-time auxiliaries in 1964; and since Table 3-6 indicates an increase in patient visits over time within categories of number of auxiliaries employed, the "percent capacity" for years before 1958 (in the case of 3 auxiliaries) and before 1970 (in the case of 4 auxiliaries) is most likely understated, in terms of the maximum visits that were actually possible in each of those years.

Proposals have been made at different times for increasing the supply of dentists. If we consider that there were, on the average, 2,400 visits per dentist (Table 3-6), then a proposed addition of 10,000 dentists to the supply of dentists would add approximately 24,000,000 potential visits to the available supply of the industry. Alternately, this increase in supply of visits could have been achieved by increasing the productivity of the existing supply of dentists by 7.5 percent in 1964. By 1970, it would have required an increase in productivity of about 6 percent. Achieving an increase in supply of visits under these alternatives, certainly differs both in cost and in timing.

The effect of increases in productivity on a greater supply of dental visits can perhaps be demonstrated when we consider that the same increase in dental visits in one year can be achieved by a 2 to 3 percent increase in productivity as by the entire graduating class from dental school. When the objective is to achieve an increase in the supply of dental services, then unless there are other goals not explicitly stated, it would appear that an evaluation of alternatives, including an analysis of the alternative use of the funds used in achieving these different programs, should be considered.

The sources from which the funds would be raised in order to finance such supply increases might also differ. Presumably Federal funds will be used to increase the supply of dentists while increases in dental productivity might be internally financed by the dental "firm" itself. An alternative use of the Federal funds might be to achieve increases in the demand for dental services. Based upon Table 3-6, projections were made of the available supply of dental services to 1975. Table 3-15 also shows the percent of the capacity of the industry that would presumably be used during the forecast period.[19]

To summarize this section on the supply of dental services, there have been large increases in dental productivity over time and a possible reason for increased use of auxiliaries is the increased demand for dental services. The ability to further increase future productivity will depend not only on continued increases in demand but also on the extent to which the dentist will be able to continue to delegate tasks to lesser skilled personnel. Some implications from

Table 3-15. Unused Capacity to Provide Dental Services, Based on Maximum Utilization of Full-Time Auxiliary Personnel, 1975

Assumption: low income and low population in 1975[1]

Year	Total Patient Visits[3]	Total Possible Visits 3 Auxiliaries per Dentist[4]	Percent Capacity[5]	Total Possible Visits 4 Auxiliaries per Dentist[4]	Percent Capacity[5]
1975	461,048,500	507,537,232	90.8	715,608,940	64.4

Assumption: high income and high population in 1975[2]

Year	Total Patient Visits[3]	Total Possible Visits 3 Auxiliaries per Dentist[4]	Percent Capacity[5]	Total Possible Visits 4 Auxiliaries per Dentist[4]	Percent Capacity[5]
1975	476,450,375	507,537,232	93.9	715,608,940	66.6

1. 1975 per capita income = $4,281; 1975 population = 213,800,000.

2. 1975 per capita income = $4,510; 1975 population = 218,000,000.

3. These figures were generated during a simulation of the Health Professions Educational Assistance program using an econometric model of the dental care sector. The reader is referred to the section on the model for an explanation of the simulation. The 1975 "low income and population" visit estimate compares favorably with an earlier estimate made by projecting the 1961-1967 rate of increase of dental visits to 1975.

4. Calculation: Active practicing dentists in year x times mean annual patient visits per dentist of dentists employing y auxiliaries. The "active practicing dentists" figure was generated during the econometric model simulation, as explained in footnote 3 above. The "visits per dentist" figure is the average of visits per dentist of dentists employing y auxiliaries in 1958, 1961, and 1964 (see Table 3-7). In other words, no productivity increase of the dentist-auxiliary "team" has been forecast beyond the 1958-1964; and the "total possible visits, y auxiliaries per dentist" figure is therefore probably understated in all cases.

5. Calculation: $\dfrac{\text{total patient visits in year } x}{\text{total possible visits, } y \text{ auxiliaries per dentist in year } x} \times 100$

this analysis of the supply of dental services are that in order to forecast future supplies of available dental care we must do more than merely forecast the number of dentists. Supply forecasts must incorporate estimates of the use of auxiliaries. Future supply estimates, therefore, should be in terms of available number of visits rather than in numbers of dentists.

Economic Determinants of the Long-Run Supply of Dental Services

When discussing the supply of dental services we may envisage three distinct time periods. The first is that period in which an increase in supply can come about only from an increase in the existing factor inputs working longer hours. (In this "immediate" period we consider that the supply of the factors cannot be enlarged, but each of the factors may work more hours.) Each succeeding time period allows greater flexibility in increasing supply. The "intermediate" period may be that time in which the dentist can increase the use of each of the factors – e.g., hire more auxiliaries, purchase more chairs, and adapt existing technology – other than adding new dentists themselves. The time required for output to increase in this intermediate stage is generally several years; this is the length of time generally required for the dentist to decide to increase and also to be able to use auxiliaries, and is the training time needed for more auxiliaries to become available. The supply of services is much greater over this intermediate period than in the immediate period. The "long run" is the time it takes to achieve an increase in the supply of dentists. In the long run the available supply will be greater than in either of the two previous periods. The most important factor determining the long-run supply of dental care, therefore, is the supply of dentists.

The "short-run" supply of dental services (immediate and intermediate periods) may be thought of as increases in the time worked by each factor and increases in factor inputs other than dentists themselves. The determinants of this supply would be the price people are willing to pay for that care, and the cost to the dentist of increasing the use of the various labor and nonlabor inputs. The cost of inputs and the resulting supply of services is also affected by the type of restrictions facing the dentist in how he can use auxiliaries. The more restrictions placed on tasks performed by auxiliaries the greater will be the cost of producing a given level of care and hence a smaller quantiy of care provided at a given price.

The determinants of the long-run supply of dentists consist of a number of factors, most of which have been studied and reported on in the literature.[20] Since the supply of dentists is a major determinant of the long-run supply of dental care and is subject to a great deal of public policy and financial support, the economic determinants of this supply should be examined. Although economic factors are only one determinant, and possibly not even the most important, the legislation and financing are directed toward this variable; therefore an estimate of its importance in affecting the supply of dentists and the effect that financial subsidies have had should be analyzed. The determinants of the supply of auxiliary personnel are also affected by many factors, among which are economic influences. Since both legislation and financing are directed toward increasing the supply of auxiliary persons, then an analysis of economic factors as they affect the supply of auxiliaries should be similarly examined.

An analysis of the long-run supply of dentists involves an examination of both the demand by persons for a dental education as well as the supply (and supply response) of dental educational institutions. In this last section we will discuss the demand for dental education, while in Chapter 4 we will examine the supply response by those training facilities.

In order to explain the demand for dental education, we must examine the economic value of the investment made by the prospective student in such a specialized form of training. The economic return to becoming a dentist or dental auxiliary may not be the most important determinant of the demand for such schooling; however, it is a factor relatively easy to manipulate if we wish to increase or decrease such demand and, more importantly, it is one means by which the government finances dental care. It is important, therefore, to determine the effectiveness of such a financing program.

Briefly stated, the economic value of an investment in dental education can be thought of as consisting of the following:

1. The out-of-pocket costs of being a dental student, which include tuition, books, etc.

2. The "opportunity cost" of spending time in dental school, that is, the income the student could have earned had he gone to work rather than to school

3. The future income to be derived from working as a dentist for a certain number of years

4. A discounting factor, which enables us to compare the future income and current costs of becoming a dentist with other occupations

The theory would suggest that if the "rate of return" to becoming a dentist increases relative to other occupations then we would expect a greater demand for places in dental schools. The converse would also hold true. The usefulness of such an approach lies in its ability to predict demand for dental education. Prospective students differ in their desire for economic objectives and their knowledge of the future is not perfect. However, to the extent that *some* students are affected by such economic considerations, it becomes a variable which enables us to predict demands for dental education and is also an important policy variable. If such economic considerations had absolutely no effect, then any financing programs affecting tuition payments or living costs would not affect the demand for dentistry as a profession. Further, any such educational revisions which decrease either the cost or the time required to become a dentist, hence increasing the prospective rate of return to become a dentist, would also affect the future supply of dentists depending upon how prospective students react to changes in their rate of return.

That the rate of return to entering any profession is important can be seen by the fact that over time virtually no profession has, on the average, a "negative" rate of return. For example, if a profession experiences decreased demand for its service, hence a drop in its incomes which bring it below the average rates of return which its prospective members could receive elsewhere, then we would expect a decrease in the demand by entrants to this profession relative to others. This does not mean that all prospective entrants change their mind, but enough do so that the rate of return will eventually rise to the point where it is once again comparable to the return its prospective entrants could receive elsewhere.

There have been relatively few studies which have attempted to estimate the rate of return to becoming a dentist. It was decided, therefore, to estimate the rate of return to a dental education for more recent periods.

The rates of return to a dental education as estimated are shown in Table 3-16. These estimates indicate the rate of return to a dental education (as though

Table 3-16. Rates of Return to a Dental Education, 1960-1970

Years Calculated	Without Scholarship Aid	With Scholarship Aid	Without Scholarship but a Decrease in Training Time of 1 Year	Without Scholarship but an Increase in Tuition (Tripling of Tuition)	Without Scholarship but an Increase in Dental Incomes of 10 Percent	Without Scholarship but an Increase in Foregone Income of 10 Percent
1960	17.5					
1965	24.2	25.8				
1970	24.5	26.8	31.6	17.4	29.7	22.5

Source: See Appendix for data sources.

this additional education were an investment) faced by an entering dental student at different periods of time. These rates of return are not "ex post" in that they are the rates of return that a prospective student would actually receive; they are "ex post" in that for any particular year the data used for each variable represents the actual value (or past value) for that variable. Theoretically, a prospective dental student would consider his "expected" rate of return, which would presumably differ from the actual rate of return received by dentists at the time the student makes his decision. To the extent that the current rates of return to a dental education are used by a prospective dental student as the best available data for estimating his expected rate of return, then the bias between these two estimates are decreased.

Students will also differ in their knowledge and expectations as to what their dental incomes are likely to be and also according to when they make their decision to attend dental school. Their actual rate of return will also differ according to where they locate, whether they practice longer than the average dentist, and so forth.

In addition to the expected rate of return to entering an occupation, the variance of the distribution of that rate of return might also be an important determinant of occupational choice. Data on the distribution of incomes of non-salaried dentists for each of the years in the ADA's *Survey of Dental Practice* suggest a relatively narrow distribution of net incomes.

For simplicity, and (primarily) because of lack of data, the calculations of rates of return implicitly assume that there are no differences in the time stream of earnings between dentists and college graduates and that the net income differences in each year are the same. Actually, it takes time for a dentist to build a practice; his income is greater in later years, and his working life may not be similar to that of the average college graduate.

There are, of course, limitations to the data used in constructing these estimates and these are indicated in Appendix 3B. The rate of return to a dental education has been persistently positive for some time. These persistently high rates of return suggest that we would expect to observe increased numbers of applicants to dental schools over time — which has, in fact, happened.

Federal legislation attempts to increase the supply of dental manpower by affecting the rate of return to prospective dentists and by subsidizing dental schools. It is important to determine the effect of subsidies to dental students in order to know how effective this legislation will be in creating more dental students or a different type of student. (The subsidy program to dental schools is discussed in Chapter 4.)

In order to estimate the effectiveness of subsidies to dental students, the sensitivity of the rate of return to several of its components was determined. As shown in Table 3-16, the rate of return to dental education was calculated for 1965 and 1970 for those students that received scholarships. The change in the rate of return for those receiving scholarships was slight. In 1965 it increased from 24.2 to 25.8, while in 1970 when more students were receiving scholarships, each of a larger amount, the rate of return only went from 24.5 to 26.8. Since another purpose of the scholarship program might have been to change the mix of students, this aspect of the subsidy program is also discussed in the next chapter.

Additional calculations were made showing the sensitivity of the rate of return to changes in any one of its components. One of these was the assumption that dental students would be charged their full costs of education as part of their tuition. In other words, dental schools would not need to receive operating subsidies if they were to pass on to students their full costs of education. It was esimated that this policy would *triple* tuition costs. If this occurred, the rate of return would decline from 24.5 to 17.4. A threefold increase in tuition costs would decrease the rate of return by several percentage points, but it would still be a good investment. For those students unable to afford the increased out-of-pocket costs of this policy, a loan program would ease the burden.

It has often been said that the dentist is overtrained for the tasks he performs. If his educational time in dental school could be reduced from four years to three, what would be the impact on the student's rate of return? In 1970, the rate of return would increase from 24.5 to 31.6 if dental education could be reduced by one year. Under such a policy we would expect to observe an even greater number of applicants to dental schools.

Two additional calculations were made describing the sensitivity of the rate of return to a change in one of its components: an increase in future dental incomes and an increase in foregone earnings. A 10 percent increase in future dental incomes would increase the rate of return from 24.5 to 29.7, while a 10 percent increase in foregone earnings while in dental school would decrease the rate of return from 24.5 to 22.5.

Since it is likely that dental incomes will continue to rise in the future as a result of the many factors affecting the demand for dental care discussed earlier, higher rates of return to dental education are likely to persist, if not increase. Such increased dental incomes will, we believe, more than offset increased tuition costs and increases in foregone earnings.

To conclude, we have seen that there are continual and persistently high rates of return to a dental education, and that current scholarship programs will make only marginal changes in these rates of return. If we assume that the alternative investment opportunity for a college graduate would be 10-15 percent, then passing the full costs of education on to the student in terms of higher tuition costs will decrease his rate of return but it will still be a worthwile investment. Shortening the educational requirements will sharply increase the rate of return, as will projected future increases in dental incomes.

If an important determinant of the future supply of dentists is the rate of return, how is it possible to explain the small increments to the supply of dentists with such persistent high rates of return? Our theory would lead us to expect large increases in enrollment, and large additions to the overall number of dentists, until the rate of return was comparable to other investment opportunities open to students. In order to explain these persistently high returns and small increments in the supply of dental manpower, we must examine the market for dental education. For it is in this market that barriers might exist that prevent rates of return from serving as a determinant of the long-run supply of dentists.

Appendix 3A: Improving the Distribution of Dentists: Subsidizing In-Migration vs. Additional Dental School Capacity

According to a study by Alex R. Maurizi[1] when "absolute net migration" of dentists into a state is the dependent variable, the coefficient of the "mean net income of nonsalaried dentists at beginning of period" is .02285 for the period 1958-1962. This relationshp makes it possible to calculate the increase in mean annual income, and therefore the per dentist subsidy, which would be necessary to attract dentists to migrate into a state:

Δ Absolute net migration of DDS = .02285 X (mean net income of dentists at beginning of period)

Therefore,

Required Δ mean net income of dentists =

$$\frac{\Delta \text{ Desired absolute net migration of DDS}}{.02285}$$

In order to have comparable cost estimates for the "migration subsidy" and "new dental school capacity" approaches, it will be assumed that 40 additional dentists are desired. (The reason for selecting 40 will be discussed below; basically, adding dentists by construction of new school capacity requires expansion by indivisible "blocks" of dentists.) Using Maruizi's coefficients, it is thus possible to calculate the cost to the state of attracting (through migration) 40 additional dentists over the period 1958-1962.

For a state to attract 40 additional dentists, dental income in that state would have to be increased by $1,750.54. ($1,750.54 is derived by dividing Maurizi's coefficient of .02285 into "absolute net migration," when "absolute net migration" equals 40, and calculating the necessary change in "mean net income.") Therefore, to attract 40 additional dentists by 1962, a state would have had to begin increasing each in-migrating dentist's income by $1,750.54 starting in 1958. Assuming that the subsidization program was aimed at young dentists with an expected remaining working life of 30 years, the total cost to the state over that time period would be $2,100,648 for 40 additional dentists ($1,750.54 x 40 dentists x 30 years). If a lump sum payment was made to each entering dentist, the present value of the annual payments would be $1.4 million dollars or $35,000 to each in-migrant (using a 5 per cent discount rate).

If the state were to subsidize the incomes of only those dentists that migrate into the state, there could conceivably be a political problem in that currently residing dentists might also wish to receive such an annual bonus. In order to resolve such an issue, the state might in fact offer a migrating dentist a lump sum subsidy equal to the present value of the annual payments, for the purpose of assisting him in establishing a practice. This subsidy could be similar to loan forgiveness programs in that the subsidy would be forgiveable if the dentist practiced a certain number of years in that state.

Alternatively, a state desiring to increase its supply of dentists over the next four years might consider building new dental school capacity and financing the education of new dental students. Between 1965 and 1971, 1,123 new dental school places were constructed at a total development cost of $345,577,920 or at an average capital cost per place of $307,727.[2] If it is assumed that a new "place" will have a useful life of 40 years, over which time it will "produce" 40 additional dentists, then the construction costs per new dentist are $7,693.

The instructional "cost of education" of a dental student for four years is approximately $30,000. (This is based on a yearly tuition figure for 1970 of $2,250, which represents about 30 percent of the total yearly "cost of education.")[3] Thus, the total cost of adding one dentist through dental school additions would be $37,693.

There can, however, be additions or subtractions to this cost. If the student paid his own tuition, which is assumed to be equal to 30 percent of his educational (instructional) costs, instead of receiving scholarship aid from the state for that amount, the cost to the state government could be reduced by up to $9,000 per graduating student. The total 40-year cost to the state will vary according to the percentage of student tuition charges paid by the state:

Percent of Tuition Charges Paid by State	Tuition Cost to State per Student per Year	Total Tuition Cost to State per Student (Over His Training Period)	Total Forty-Year Cost to State of Developing Forty New Dentists
100%	$2250	$9000	$1,508,000
67%	$1500	$6000	$1,388,000
50%	$1125	$4500	$1,328,000
33%	$ 750	$3000	$1,268,000
0%	$ 0	$ 0	$1,148,000

Further, matching fund support for dental school construction is available under the HPEA program; in the 1965-1971 period this support averaged $154,252 per new school place constructed.[4] Assuming an output per place of 40 dentists, this federal subsidy would lower the cost to the state by $3,856 per new dentist. Additional support coming from foundations, philanthropic groups, federal grants, etc., would further lower the costs to the state.

On the other hand, in constructing a new dental school place, the state cannot just spend $7,693 to build space for one more student; it must spend the entire construction cost of $307,727 per place, and thus purchase an indivisible "block" of 40 additional dentists, to be produced at the rate of one per year over the next 40 years. If the state were to subsidize the entire cost (instructional as well as capital costs) of each student's dental education, then the total 40-year cost to the state for producing 40 additional dentists, would be approximately $1,508,000 (construction expenses of $307,727, plus cost of education subsidies of $30,000 per dentist times 40 dentists, assuming no cost increases in provision of instructional services over the 40-year period). When the instructional costs are discounted ($600,000) and added to the outlay for construction costs, the total outlay for the state would be $908,000.

The "new dental school capacity method" cost of $908,000 can thus be compared to the "migration-subsidy method" cost of $1,400,000. However, while each of these figures represents the cost of adding 40 additional dentists to the state's supply, they are still not completely comparable. In addition to using cost data for different time periods with the "new school capacity method," the additional dentists are supplied at a rate of one per year for 40 years, whereas in the latter method, all 40 dentists are supplied within four years. Therefore the migration method will result in an additional dentist today rather than having an additional dentist x years from today. It should be remembered that although the "new dental school capacity method" will produce 40 additional dental school graduates, not all of these will necessarily practice in the same state in which they were trained. In fact, national statistics show that a large percentage of dentists are practicing in states other than the one in which they graduated from dental school.[5]

Those areas of the nation which most need dentists (and thus would be most interested in attracting in-migrating dentists with subsidies) are more likely to lose their "new dental school" graduates through out-migration. The fact that a large percentage of the 40 new graduates that a state would produce through building new school capacity would leave that state, will significantly raise the "average cost" of producing a new dentist in this manner. For example, in 1970 only 46.2 percent of the graduates of dental schools in the southeast region (Alabama, Arkansas, Florida, Georgia, Kentucky, Louisiana, Mississippi, North Carolina, South Carolina, Tennessee, Virginia) were practicing in the same state in which they were trained. This means that of 40 dentists graduated from schools in a particular southeastern state, only about eighteen would establish practice in that state.

To produce 40 new dentists that remain in the state via the "new dental school capacity method" would require 87 graduates for a total cost of $2,000,000 in present value as compared to $1,400,000 for the cash payment program.

Alternatively, the typical southeastern area state might want to compare the cost of producing eighteen additional dentists over 40 years (which given the expected out-migration of dental school graduates, would require providing dental school capacity and financial support for 40 graduates over 40 years), versus the cost of attracting eighteen additional in-migrating dentists through subsidization. Again using Maurizi's coefficient of .02285, the yearly per-dentist subsidy necessary to attract eighteen additional migrants will be $787.75.

Continuing the assumption that in-migrating dentists would be relatively young and thus have a relatively long expected remaining working life of 30 years, over which they would be paid the yearly subsidy, the total cost to the state of "migration-subsidy method" now becomes $425,385 ($787.75 X 18 dentists X 30 years) and when discounted is equal to $245,500. This compares with the cost of the "new dental school capacity method" (which remains the same) of $908,000 to produce eighteen additional dentists over 40 years.

This example of the relative costs to the state for increasing its number of dentists by subsidizing dentists to migrate to that state, as compared to increasing its dental school capacity, should be considered illustrative of the type of analysis that should be undertaken for such a decision; the data used were aggregate and in some instances were for different time periods. Also no allowance was made for the differences in time during which new dentists would be available when the method of increasing dental school capacity was used.

Appendix 3B. Rates of Return Calculated by A. Maurizi and W. Hansen

There have been two other studies that have calculated rates of return to a dental education. W. Hansen and A. Maurizi calculated their rates of return by finding the rate of discount that equates "the present value of the expected earnings stream to the present values of the expected outlay or cost stream" (Hansen) and "the present value of costs to the present value of returns" (Maurizi), where "returns" indicates the difference between the earnings of dentists and the earnings of the selected population.

There are a number of differences between these two studies, the main one is that Hansen compares the cost and benefit of entering dentistry to that of going to work upon graduation from high school. Thus his return stream consists of the difference between the earnings of practicing dentists and those of male high school graduates; and his training costs include those of the undergraduate education. Maurizi's study (and ours) calculates the difference in returns between dentists and college graduates. This difference in the base population is probably the main reason for the difference in magnitude between Hansen's and Maurizi's rates of return, as shown below.

Year	Hansen[1]	Maurizi[2,3]
1939	12.3	
1948		19.1
1949	13.4	
1952		21.0
1955		18.5
1956	12.0	
1958		14.8
1961		17.9

Sources:

[1] W. Lee Hansen, "Shortages and Investment in Health Manpower," in *The Economics of Health and Medical Care*, Proceedings of the Conference on the Economics of Health and Medical Care, May 10-12, 1962, The University of Michigan, Ann Arbor, Michigan, 1969, p. 86.

[2] Zero draft probability assumption.

[3] Alex Maurizi, "Rates of Return in the Dental Profession," *Economic Essays on the Dental Profession*, College of Business Administration, The University of Iowa, Iowa City, Iowa, 1969, p. 13.

There are a number of other differences in methodology among the three studies. For example, in Hansen's calculations, earnings of the dental student during the training period are not subtracted from costs, as they are in the other two studies. Maurizi's calculations differ from the other calculations in the subtraction of the student wife's earnings from training costs. He also introduces mortality probabilities for each age group, and draft assumptions (percentage chance of being drafted) for both graduated dentists and men with college degrees. An important difference between both the Hansen and Maurizi studies and ours was that Hansen and Maurizi used cross sectional data to determine dental earnings at every age for each year of calculation, then used these age bracket earnings to construct an expected stream of earnings over the dentist's lifetime.

In our study the rate of return is that rate of discount that equates the present value of the differences between mean annual dentist income and mean annual income of the college graduate to the present value of (discounted) costs of dental training. Since mean annual income data was more readily available than cross sectional age bracket data, this method enabled us to calculate rates of return for a greater number of years. Because of these differences, and others, we would expect the rates of return in all three studies to differ. However, since Hansen's study calculated the rate of return from the point of view of high school graduates, his estimates would be less comparable to ours than Maurizi's.

In addition to the rates of return shown in Table 3-16, we made similar calculations for 1940, 1950, and 1955, which were 18.8, 15.5, and 22.8 respectively. These differ from Maurizi's in that his rate of return for 1948 was 19.1 as compared to ours of 15.5 in 1950; 18.5 (Maurizi) versus 22.8 in 1955; and 17.9 in 1961 versus 17.5 for 1960. Although there are differences between these two series, a similar pattern exists. Rates of return increased in the post World War II period until the 1950s (1952 – Maurizi, 1955 – our series), they then declined until the end of that decade (1958 – Maurizi, 1960 – our series) and then continued their rise in the 1960s (1961 – Maurizi, 1965 – our series).

The main purpose of this discussion has been to demonstrate that despite differences in methodology and in the actual estimates of the rates of return, (1) the rate of return to a dental education has been consistently positive and high since the post World War II period – all three studies agree on this – and (2) the rate of return appears to be sufficiently large so that a sensitivity analysis of the 1970 rate of return indicates the economic feasibility of having dental students bear a larger portion of their costs of education.

Appendix 3C. Definition of Variables, Data Sources, and Calculations for Estimating Rates of Return to a Dental Education

The rate of return (shown in Table 3-16) is that rate of discount which equates the difference between the mean annual income of dentists and the mean annual income of college graduates to the discounted costs of dental education. These costs consist of tuition, fees, and equipment costs paid by the student; plus the earnings foregone by the student while in dental school (measured as the average starting salary of college graduates); lessened by the average value of income earned by dental students through term time and summer employment. This differs somewhat from the more traditional method of using a stream of returns over the dentist's working life.

Rates of return under several other assumptions were also calculated. To measure the rate of return to entering dental school with scholarship aid, the rate was recalculated for 1965 and 1970 with the educational expenses lessened by the average value of scholarship awards in those years. To measure the effects of reducing dental training time to three years, the rate of return was calculated for 1970, using educational expenses, foregone earnings, and actual earnings for only three years. Another rate of return for 1970 was calculated with tuition expenses increased threefold, to represent the cost of charging the dental student the entire cost of his education. To determine the effects of an increased average dentist income, the rate was recalculated for 1970 with "Mean Annual Income of Dentists" increased by 10 percent. Finally, to measure the effects of a higher starting salary for college graduates, the rate of return was recalculated for 1970 with "foregone earnings" increased by 10 percent. The formula used for all calculations is, with modifications as indicated:

$$r = \frac{\text{Mean Annual Income of Dentist (1-Tax Rate)} - \text{Mean Annual Income of College Graduate (1-Tax Rate)}}{\sum_{i=1}^{4} \dfrac{\text{Costs}}{(1 + \text{Corporate Bond Rate})^{i-1}}}$$

Data Sources for Appendix 3C
(The actual data will be provided upon request)

1. *Mean Annual Income of Dentists*

Sources: William Weinfeld, *Survey of Current Business,* January 1950 for the period before 1950, and American Dental Association, *Survey of Dental Practice,* 1956, 1959, 1962, 1965, 1968, *JADA,* February 1972.

2. *Mean Annual Income of College Graduates (All Ages)*

Sources: *U.S. Historical Statistics,* p. 97; *1940 Census of Population, Education,* "Educational Attainment by Economic Characteristics," Tables 29 and 31; *1950 Census of Population,* Series P-E, No. 5B Education, Tables 12 and 13; *Current Population Survey,* Consumer Income Supplements, March 1959; *Current Population Survey,* Consumer Income, p. 27, Table 7, Education of Head-Families and Unrelated Individuals by Total Money Income in 1964, by Years of School Completed — Median Income; Katona, George, Lewis Mandell, and Jay Schmideskamp. *1970 Survey of Consumer Finances,* Survey Research Center, Institute for Social Research, University of Michigan, Ann Arbor, Michigan, 1971, p. 12; *Statistical Abstract of the U.S.,* 1965; Miller, Herman P., "Annual and Lifetime Income in Relation to Education: 1939-1959," *American Economic Review* (December 1960), pp. 962-985, Table 1; *Current Population Survey* Consumer Income Supplements, March 1947 and April 1947.

3. *Income Tax Rates*

Sources: *U.S. Historical Statistics,* p. 716 and 1962 Supplement for 1930-1960; Tax Foundation, Inc., *Facts and Figures on Government Finance,* 13th edition, 1964-1965, p. 104; 1971 Tax Form 1040, Tables p. 18.

4. *Basic Yield of Corporate Bonds with 20-Year Maturities*

Sources: *U.S. Historical Statistics; Statistical Abstract of the U.S.,* 1971, p. 446.

5. *Average Value of Dental Scholarship Awards*

Sources: *Hearings Before the Committee on Interstate and Foreign Commerce, House of Representatives,* 87th Congress, Second Session, on H.R. 4999, H.R. 8774, and H.R. 8833, January 23, 24, 25, 26, and 30, 1962 — supplementary statement on the American Dental Association, p. 182 — U.S. Government Printing Office, Washington, D.C., 1962; *Hearings Before the Subcommittee on Public Health and Environment of the Committee on Interstate and Foreign Commerce, House of Representatives,* 92nd Congress, 1st Session, on H.R. 703, 4171, 4155, 5614, 5767, 7765, 4145, 4156, 4618, 7707, 7736, April 2, 3, 20, 21, 22, 23, 27, 28, 29, 1971 — statement of Dr. James W. Bowden, Dean, University of North Carolina School of Dentistry, in behalf of the American Dental Association and American Association of Dental Schools — accompanied by Dr. Richard K. Mosbaugh, Chairman, Council on Legislation, ADA and Hal M. Christensen, Director, Washington Office, ADA, U.S. Government Printing Office, Washington, D.C. 1971, p. 74.

6. *Tuition and Fee Expenses of Dental Students*

Sources: University of Michigan, School of Dentistry *Announcement;* Figure used is a weighted average of in-state and out-of-state tuition rates (in-state = .68, out-of-state = .32; see Alex Maurizi, "Rates of Return in the Dental

Profession," in *Economic Essays on the Dental Profession,* College of Business Administration, The University of Iowa, Iowa City, Iowa, 1969, p. 28) plus .8125 of tuition charges to account for equipment and other learning expenses (ratio derived from information given in *Hearings Before the Committee on Interstate and Foreign Commerce, House of Representatives,* 87th Congress, Second Session, on H.R. 4999, H.R. 8774, and H.R. 8833, June 23, 24, 25, 26, and 30, 1962 Summary Statement of the American Dental Association, U.S. Government Printing Office, Washington, D.C., 1962, p. 179); American Association of Dental Schools, *Cost Study of Dental Education 1963-1964,* Chapel Hill, N.C., 1965, p. 20 (figure used is an average yearly tuition charges in 45 reporting dental schools, plus .8125 of tuition charges to account for equipment and other learning expenses, as explained under 1930 data above; *Hearings Before the Subcommittee on Public Health and Environment of the Committee on Interstate and Foreign Commerce, House of Representatives,* 92nd Congress, 1st Session, on H.R. 703, 4171, 4155, 5614, 4767, 7765, 4145, 4156, 4618, 7707, 7736, April 2, 3, 20, 21, 22, 23, 27, 28, 29, 1971 – statement of Dr. James W. Bowden, Dean, University of North Carolina School of Dentistry, in behalf of the American Dental Association and American Association of Dental Schools – accompanied by Dr. Richard K. Mosbaugh, Chairman, Council on Legislation, ADA, and Hal M. Christensen, Director, Washington Office, ADA, U.S. Government Printing Office, Washington, D.C., 1971, p. 717.

7. *Income Foregone By Dental Student During Training* (Starting Salary of College Graduate)

Sources: Schultz, Theodore, "Capital Formation by Education," *Journal of Political Economics,* December 1960, p. 580; *Reader's Digest Almanac,* 1966, p. 385; University of Michigan Placement Service, from College Placement Council, *Salary Survey,* July 1971.

8. *Average Annual Earnings of Dental Student During Training*

Source: Figures are derived by applying ratios of .033 (to determine term-time earnings) and .0134 (to determine summer earnings) to the mean annual income of dentists for year x. Ratios derived from relationship between term-time earnings and mean annual income of dentists for 1953, and between summer earnings and mean annual income of dentists for 1960. See Alex Maurizi, "Rates of Return in the Dental Profession," *Economic Essays on the Dental Profession,* College of Business Administration, University of Iowa, Iowa City, Iowa, 1969, p. 27.

The Demand for and Supply of Educational Facilities in the Dental Sector

One of the submarkets in the dental care sector is the educational market — that is, where dentists and hygienists are trained. An analysis of this market is important for two reasons: first, since government funds are used to subsidize part of this market a question naturally arises as to the effect of such subsidies, should such subsidies be increased or could they be better spent in another part of the dental care sector? The second reason for examining this sector is that the performance of this market has a direct bearing on the long-run price and quantity of dental care available.

While the discussion in the chapter on supply of dental services was concerned primarily with the short-run supply response to increased demand for dental services, an understanding of the dental education sector is necessary for determining the long-run supply response. For example, if there was a large increase in the number of dentists and hygienists, then this would result in an increase in the availability (supply) of dental care. Similarly, changes in the supply of dentists would have an important effect on future changes in the price of dental care. Because we are interested in the price of dental care and the quantity used by various population groups, it becomes necessary to analyze the structure of the education market in order to evaluate its performance and the implications of government financing in this area.

The supply of dental education consists of two major parts, the more important being the educational training for dentists. The other training facilities are for three allied occupational groups: dental hygienists, dental assistants, and dental laboratory technicians. As with an economic analysis of any market, the educational market for dentists and dental auxiliaries should be examined in terms of the determinants of demand for training at such educational institutions, and on the supply side, the determinants of the supply of such educational institutions and the resultant number of places for training. Knowledge of these underlying factors will enable us to predict the number of graduates from known changes in either demand or supply factors.

Determinants of the Demand for Dental Education and Dental Auxiliaries

There are of course many factors that influence a person's choice to become a dentist or a dental auxiliary, and the importance of each of these factors probably varies with each individual. However, as discussed in the section on

105

rates of return to a dental education, the income potential or the economic value of that education to the student is important. This demand determinant — the rate of return to a dental education — was found to be persistently positive throughout the post-World War II period. It was concluded therefore that the reason for not having more dentists was not for a lack of demand by persons to becoming dentists.

That there was (and still is) a sufficient demand for dental education can also be seen by looking at data on the number of applicants and acceptances to dental schools. As shown in Table 4-1, the percent of applicants enrolled is less

Table 4-1. Dental School Applicants: 1955-1956 and 1960-1961 through 1969-1970

Academic Year	Dental School Applicants	First-year Dental Students	Applicants per Student Enrolled	Percent of Applicants Enrolled
1955-1956	7,205	3,445	2.1	48
1960-1961	6,119	3,616	1.7	59
1961-1962	5,841	3,605	1.6	62
1962-1963	6,566	3,680	1.8	56
1963-1964	8,969	3,770	2.4	42
1964-1965	9,598	3,836	2.5	40
1965-1966	9,988	3,806	2.6	38
1966-1967	10,177	3,942	2.6	39
1967-1968	10,264	4,200	2.4	41
1968-1969	9,037	4,203	2.2	46
1969-1970	10,325	4,355	2.4	42

Source: American Dental Association, Council on Dental Education. Applicants to Dental School 1967 and previous years (unpublished).

Published in *Manpower Supply and Educational Statistics for Dentists and Dental Auxiliaries,* P.H.S., publication No. 263, section 20 (as of March 1971), p. 40.

than half. (The data in Table 4-1 on "Dental School Applicants" are on the number of persons applying for admission to one or more dental schools each year, *not* the number of applications.) Further, this low ratio of acceptances is not a temporary phenomenon but is persistent and is even getting lower. It must be concluded therefore that the small annual increase in number of dental school graduates is not a result of a lack of demand by entrants for this profession, for from 1955 to 1970 the average annual percent increase in dental school graduates has been 1.76.

Any governmental financing program therefore that has as its goal an increased number of dental graduates and hopes to achieve this objective by subsidizing the dental student will meet with little success. We would expect such a program will increase the demand for dental education (since this would increase the rate of return), a higher number of applicants to dental schools will result, with a consequent *smaller* percent of applicants enrolled by the schools.

It may be said that the "quality" of the accepted dental student will be higher since the school will be able to be more selective in meeting its quota. It is dubious, though, that the measures of quality employed by the school are perfect indicators of performance for a working dentist. However, the more important objection to restriction of entrants in order to increase "quality" of prospective dentists is the notion that with a smaller supply of dentists some persons will go without dental care at all and that those who do receive it will probably be paying a higher price and not receive as much as if there were a greater availability of dentists.

The measurement of "quality" should not just be based upon the qualifications of the entering student, nor even solely on the quality of care received by a patient. Rather a more comprehensive index should be considered which would weigh those who do not receive any dental care because there is an inadequate supply as well as those persons who do receive dental care. The trade-off between the requirements for producing high quality dental care and the consequent smaller supply of dentists, with the result that many do not receive any care at all, is an important consideration. Most professionals, however, will opt for very high quality for those who can afford it.

With regard to the demand for educational training by dental auxiliaries, there is some evidence to suggest that the demand for such training has greatly increased in recent years. The salaries of dental auxiliaries have been increasing relative to salaries paid in oceupations with roughly comparable requirements. The relative wage of dental assistants to that of secretaries, stenographers, and typists was .81 in 1955. (Median salary of a dental assistant in 1955 was $2,333 while for a secretary, stenographer, and typist it was $2,877.) In 1971, although salaries of both groups increased, salaries for dental assistants increased more rapidly so that their relative wage was now 1.06 (the salaries were now $4,764 and $4,494).[1] When other occupational groups are used, for example workers employed in the retail trade, the same relationship is evident. The relative wage was .72 in 1950 and 1.11 in 1971. This large increase in the wages of dental assistants relative to other occupations suggests that there has been an increase in the demand for dental assistants. Although the majority of dental assistants receive on-the-job training, increased standards for certification for dental assisting would (depending upon its affect on the rate of return) increase the demand for the formal educational requirements in order to meet those standards.[2] It is also possible to make some inferences on the market structure for auxiliary training and its performance when we next examine the supply response by their educational institutions.

The Supply Response of Training Facilities for Dentists and Dental Auxiliaries

When the demand for dental education was discussed above, it was said that one factor affecting this demand was the relative rate of return to becoming a dentist. And that changes in any of the components of this rate of return would produce a change in the demand for dental education. However, when we discuss the determinants of the supply of such educational spaces, we run into difficulty if we use a similar economics variable. The reason is obvious; the objective of dental schools is not to maximize profit nor even to make money. These are the traditional incentives that cause institutions and firms to respond to increased demands for their products or services.

If the market for dental schools was organized in a competitive framework, with a similar set of incentives, then supply would respond to increases in demand and, second, the supply would be produced in a least cost manner (for a given level of quality). Let us examine the dental school sector according to both of these "ideal" criteria.

If dental schools were to respond in the traditional manner as would a competitive industry to increased demand, then it would work something like this: observing an increase in applicants, dental schools would, in the short run, have to ration their spaces as they are currently doing. However, if they perceive that this increased demand will continue, they will start to attract additional faculty, staff, equipment, and physical space. The effect on their average cost per student of this expansion (assuming, for simplicity, no external dis-economies) will depend on whether they are currently small so that they can benefit from economies of scale, meaning that as they expand, the cost of training additional students is less than the previous average, thus leading to lower average training costs. However, when a certain size has been achieved, their average cost per student will begin to increase because of increased administration costs, the lowering of teaching quality as class sizes become too large, lack of coordination, and so forth.

Under these circumstances – i.e., a normal response to increased demand – the expansion of dental school capacity would occur among schools that were previously smaller than the optimum size, and in the construction of new dental schools. As the profession expands, dental incomes will begin to fall relative to other occupations, and the rate of return to becoming a dentist will decline, until the rate is normal. Investment in and expansion of dental school capacity will then begin to slow down as more students become dentists.

Further, if dental schools were to operate in a manner similar to a perfectly competitive market, then tuition charges would reflect the full costs of educating a dental student. Tuition would then serve the same functions that prices do in such markets. As applied to the dental education market these functions would be as follows.

Incentives Toward Internal Efficiency

There are a number of factors that affect educational costs per student between schools. Several of the more important of these are the efficiency of the educational process, the scale at which the school operates, and the quality of instruction it provides. As long as subsidies are available, tuition charges can be maintained artificially low and a school that would have higher costs per student because it is either less efficient or operates at too small a size is not penalized. Without subsidies such schools would be forced to lower their costs per student (if a student can select among comparable schools with much lower tuition charges) or face a decrease in their demand and eventually go out of business. With regard to higher costs because of differences in quality of instruction, there would be demands by students for different levels of quality education (as currently exists for undergraduate and graduate education) and these quality differences would be priced accordingly. Thus the amount of quality produced (and the different levels) would be determined not by the schools, as is currently the practice, but by student demand.

Opposition to such a proposal on the grounds that students are not sufficiently knowledgeable regarding choices on quality of schools and tuition charges would suggest a policy that each school should attempt to make these differences more explicit to potential applicants. There would always be the fear among dental schools that differences in tuition between schools reflect more than differences in quality. Making these costs explicit and comparing them to other schools would always be embarrassing to those schools below the mean.

The Allocation Between Public and Private Institutions

Currently, publicly supported dental schools have, on the average, higher per student costs than do private dental schools. However, because public dental schools are more heavily subsidized, they are able to charge lower tuition rates than private schools. The effect of this is to cause a shift in the education of dentists toward public institutions and to jeopardize the financial status of the private dental schools or those relying more heavily on tuition charges. (An additional consequence would be a lowering of the quality of the education in those schools with lower per student subsidies.)[3] If, however, tuition were to reflect the full cost of education in each institution, then the selection of dental schools by students would be based in part on their relative costs and their reputation for quality of education.

The Optimal Quantity of Dental Education

If tuition did reflect the full cost of a dental education, and the supply of such education was to respond to changes in tuition rates, then the calculation of rates of return to a dental education would more accurately reflect the value to society of that education. (This assumes no external benefits nor imperfections in the market for dental education. A more complete discussion of external benefits and imperfections in the markets for capital and risk bearing is postponed until Chapter 6.)

In addition to determining the optimal quantity of dental education, tuition rates would also determine the optimal distribution of dental outputs within each school (and similarly for all dental schools). It presumably cost the school different amounts to produce dentists, dental specialists, etc. If these differences in costs between dental school outputs were reflected in different tuition charges, then the demand for such training would be affected, hence the quantity of these specialties produced. Since tuition does not currently reflect the full costs of dental education, it does not serve as an incentive for schools to minimize their costs, to operate at the least cost size, nor to produce the optimal amount of dental education. Without such a price mechanism, how can we be sure that these desirable outcomes are achieved?

The current pricing policy of dental schools cannot be justified on grounds of redistribution of income, since it is clearly inequitable. The educational subsidies are received by those students whose families have relatively higher family incomes. If it were desired to subsidize students of low income families to become dentists, it would be more efficient to subsidize such students directly rather than provide subsidies to all students by subsidizing schools to lower their tuition charges. The supply response of training facilities for dental auxiliaries is different from that of dental schools and appears to be similar to a more freely operating market.

Table 4-2. Number of Schools, Students, and Graduates in the Field of Dental Assisting in the United States: Academic Years 1961-1962 through 1969-1970

Academic Year	Number of Dental Assistants		
	Schools	Students	Graduates
1961-1962	26	1,181	658
1962-1963[1]	33	1,419	718
1963-1964	40	1,551	895
1964-1965	50	1,919	1,241
1965-1966	64	2,798	1,593
1966-1967	81	3,159	1,963
1967-1968	101	3,819	2,302
1968-1969	134	4,475	2,715
1969-1970	153	5,074	—

1. Figures for 1962-1963 and thereafter, include the University of Puerto Rico, its dental assistant students and graduates.

Source: American Dental Association, Council on Dental Education. Unpublished data from Dental Students' Register Questionnaire for 1961-1962, and Dental Students' Register, 1962-1963 through 1966-1967.

American Dental Association, Council on Dental Education. Annual Report on Dental Auxiliary Education, 1967-1968, 1968-1969 and 1969-1970.

Published in *Manpower Supply and Educational Statistics for Dentists and Dental Auxiliaries,* PHS publication No. 263 Section 20. (as of March 1971). p. 41.

According to Tables 4-2, 4-3, 4-4 the market for educational training in the fields of dental assisting, dental hygiene, and dental laboratory technicians have experienced very large increases in capacity to provide such training and their output of graduates. In a ten-year period, the number of schools and their output have increased by approximately sixfold and fivefold respectively for dental laboratory technicians and dental assistants; while for dental hygienists, the number of schools offering such programs has tripled with an almost equal increase in their graduates. During the last ten years the number of schools for dental laboratory technicians has gone from 4 to 23 while the number of graduates from these programs has increased from 78 to 357.[4]

Thus the market for the training of dental auxiliaries appears to respond, as perhaps would a competitive industry to increases in demand for such training. Additional supplies of dental auxiliaries might therefore be more affected by

Table 4-3. Number of Schools, Students and Graduates in the Field of Dental Hygiene in the United States: Selected Academic Years 1930-1931 through 1969-1970

Academic Year	Number of Dental Hygiene Students		
	Schools	Students	Graduates
1930-1931	17	—	354
1935-1936	19	—	335
1940-1941	18	—	366
1945-1946	17	678	403
1950-1951	27	1,454	636
1955-1956	33	2,009	902
1959-1960	34	2,237	992
1960-1961	37	2,497	1,023
1961-1962	43	2,752	1,219
1962-1963	47	3,005	1,257
1963-1964	49	3,276	1,429
1964-1965	53	3,502	1,491
1965-1966	56	3,863	1,650
1966-1967	58	4,041	1,739
1967-1968	67	4,309	1,834
1968-1969	85	5,187	2,231
1969-1970[1]	100	5,931	—

1. Figures for 1969-1970 include the University of Puerto Rico, its dental hygiene students and graduates.

Source: Pelton, Walter J.; Pennell, Elliott H.; and Vaura, Helen M. Health Manpower Source Book. Dental Hygienists. Public Health Service Publication No. 263, Section 8. U.S. Government Printing Office, Washington, D.C., 1957.

American Dental Association, Council on Dental Education. Dental Students' Register, 1959-1960 through 1966-1967.

American Dental Association, Council on Dental Education. Annual Report on Dental Auxiliary Education, 1967-1968, 1968-1969 and 1969-1970.

Published in *Manpower Supply and Educational Statistics for Dentists and Dental Auxiliaries,* PHS publication No. 263, Section 20. (as of March 1971), p. 54.

Table 4-4. Number of Programs, Students and Graduates in the Field of Dental Laboratory Technology in the United States: Academic Years 1959-1960 through 1969-1970

Academic Year	Number of Dental Laboratory Technology Students		
	Programs	Students	Graduates
1959-1960	3	184	78
1960-1961	4	230	81
1961-1962	4	273	95
1962-1963	5	295	108
1963-1964	5	285	104
1964-1965	5	343	119
1965-1966	6	342	142
1966-1967	10	510	162
1967-1968	15	729	325
1968-1969	19	803	357
1969-1970	23	965	—

Source: American Dental Association, Council on Dental Education. Dental Students' Register, 1959-1960 through 1966-1967.

American Dental Association, Council on Dental Education. Annual Report on Dental Auxiliary Education, 1967-1968, 1968-1969 and 1969-1970.

Published in *Manpower Supply and Educational Statistics for Dentists and Dental Auxiliaries,* PHS publications No. 263, Section 20. (as of March 1971), p. 65.

their increased educational requirements and whether there are compensating increases in their relative wages than by the lack of available spaces for such training.

An important question, therefore, is why doesn't the output of dental graduates from dental schools also respond to increased demand for such training? During the same ten-year period the increase in dental graduates went from 3,290 to 3,500 as shown in Table 4-5 below. It thus appears that the bottleneck to increased output of dental graduates is not on the demand side but on the *supply* response by these educational institutions.

Economies of Scale in the Production of Dentists

In addition to this lack of responsiveness by dental schools to their increased demand, it also appears that this industry is not producing its output — graduates — as efficiently as possible. In order to produce dental graduates most efficiently, one important consideration is whether dental schools are taking advantage of any economies of scale that might exist. The nature of economies of scale in dental education would presumably be "U" Shaped and appear as shown in Figure 4-1, which is the theoretical relationship between average cost per student and dental school class size. Since the number of yearly graduates from different dental schools varies from 17 to 158 graduates per year, with the

Table 4-5. Number of Dental Schools, Dental Students and Dental Graduates in the United States: Selected Academic Years 1930-1931 through 1969-1970

Academic Year	Number of Dental Schools	Number of Dental Students		Number of Dental Graduates
		Total	First Year	
1930-1931	38	8,129	1,929	1,842
1935-1936	39	7,306	2,161	1,736
1940-1941	39	7,720	2,305	1,568
1945-1946	39	7,274	1,201	2,666
1950-1951	42	11,891	3,226	2,830
1955-1956	43	12,730	3,445	3,038
1960-1961[1]	47	13,580	3,616	3,290
1961-1962	47	13,513	3,605	3,207
1962-1963	48	13,576	3,680	3,233
1963-1964	48	13,691	3,770	3,213
1964-1965	49	13,876	3,836	3,181
1965-1966	49	14,020	3,806	3,198
1966-1967	49	14,421	3,942	3,360
1967-1968	50	14,955	4,200	3,457
1968-1969	52	15,408	4,203	3,433
1969-1970	53	16,008	4,355	3,500[2]

1. Figures for academic year 1960-1961 and thereafter include the University of Puerto Rico, its dental students and its dental graduates.

2. As estimated by American Dental Association.

Source: U.S. Bureau of the Census, Historical Statistics of the United States, Colonial Times to 1957, U.S. Government Printing Office, Washington, D.C. 1960.

American Dental Association, Council on Dental Education. Dental Students' Register. Required issues 1939-1940 through 1966-1967.

American Dental Association, Council on Dental Education. Annual Report on Dental Education, 1967-1968, 1968-1969 and 1969-1970, Parts 1.

Published in *Manpower Supply and Educational Statistics for Dentists and Dental Auxiliaries,* PHS publication No. 263, Section 20. (as of March 1971), p. 5.

average being 66,[5] it would appear (and as the evidence to be presented will indicate) that many schools in the industry are producing graduates at a relatively higher per unit cost than other schools because they are too small.

It seems difficult to imagine that, if quality was held constant, each of these schools was equally efficient in producing dentists from class sizes that varied so greatly. If economies of scale were to exist, then an increased number of dentists at a lower per unit cost could be achieved if the smaller schools were to increase their class sizes.

There are a number of difficulties in estimating the relationship of cost to size between dental schools. Foremost among these difficulties is the ability to hold constant the effect of differences in quality of instruction between schools. When quality of instruction is described on an input basis, we observe wide variations among schools in their use of full-time as compared to volunteer or part-time faculty, for example from 0 to 85 percent.[6] Also, differences in the

Figure 4-1. The Relationship Between Dental School Class Size and Cost per
Student

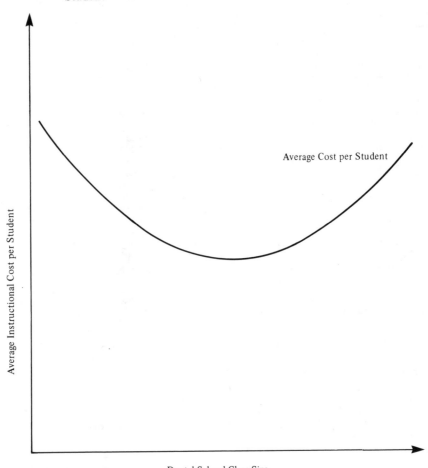

Average Cost per Student

Average Instructional Cost per Student

Dental School Class Size

amount of clinical training a student receives may be more related to its
income-generating effects on the school rather than on his future practice needs.
Differences also exist in the ratio of students to faculty and equipment in the
clinical portion of their training as well as to the degree to which there is
subsidization of student teaching by faculty supported by research funds.

If it were thus possible to isolate the true costs of instruction and control for
differences in quality and efficiency of instruction (unrelated to size), then it
would be possible to examine the effects of size and costs, which would
probably be more related to the basic sciences portion of the instruction.

These difficulties aside, however, a preliminary attempt was made to
determine the extent of economies of scale in dental education in order to

estimate the possible savings if such economies were achieved. According to Table 4-6, average cost per student declines with increased dental school enrollment. This decrease in per student costs exists for both public and private dental schools and persists over time.[7] Data on instruction cost per student in both public and private dental schools, for different time periods, were also examined through the use of multiple regression analysis. (These results are presented in Appendix 4, Table 4-A.)

The implications of possible economies of scale in the production of dentists are significant when we consider that there are alternative means of financing an increase in dental school output. One method currently employed under the Health Professions Educational Assistance Act (HPEA) is to finance both existing and new dental schools. It should be possible to achieve an additional output of graduates at a much lower cost by financing some schools rather than others. The selection of schools would depend upon where on the cost-size relationship different schools are, and where they are likely to be if they increase their output. The goals of this policy can be implemented by financing dental schools on a capitation basis — that is, relating the amount of funds to increased

Table 4-6. Average Yearly Cost of Dental Education per Student by School Size, 1964 and 1969-1970

	Enrollment					
	1-200		201-300		301+	
1964[1]	Number of Schools	Average Cost	Number of Schools	Average Cost	Number of Schools	Average Cost
Public Schools	4	$3,802	7	$3,716	8	$2,658
Private Schools	7	$3,475	9	$2,554	9	$2,070
Total Schools	11		16		17	
1969-1970[2]	1-250		251-350		351+	
Public Schools	9	$9,379	5	$9,059	10	$7,635
Private Schools	7	$6,469	6	$5,897	10	$5,160
Total Schools	16		11		20	

1. *Source:* American Association of Dental Schools, *Cost Study of Dental Education,* 1965. The figures represent the cost of the instructional program for the undergraduate dental student who is studying for the D.D.S. or D.M.D. degree, based upon the percent of effort method of analysis. The figures do not include expenditures on research, the cost of providing basic science instruction, or "indirect expenditures" (expenditures of the university as a whole a percentage of which the dental school may be "charged" in an accounting sense).

2. *Source:* American Dental Association, *The Annual Report on Dental Education 1970-1971: Financial Information.* Chicago, Illinois, 1971; plus correspondence with James Mastro, Project Director, Annual Survey of Dental Educational Institutions. The figures are for regular dental school programs, which include expenditures from the dental school budget and estimated costs of basic science instruction.

output of graduates. The capitation grant could be based upon the average cost per student in a large dental school that is considered efficient (empirical estimates of this could be derived). Unless a dental school receiving such capitation grants strove to become as large and as efficient as possible, the capitation grant would not be sufficient to cover its costs per student. For example, a school with a cost per student of $6,000 would receive a greater percentage subsidy than would a school that had a cost per student of $10,000. Such a financing mechanism would thus provide an incentive toward increased output as well as toward minimum costs per student.

The reason why dental schools have not taken advantage of economies of scale in dental education and why they have not responded to increased demand for their spaces (as have the educational facilities for dental auxiliaries) are probably related. The goals and incentives facing dental schools must be better understood if subsidies to these schools are to result in an increased number of graduates. For unless such schools are more responsive to their increased demands, then government financing of schools, both existing and new ones, without any incentives tied to such grants, will merely perpetuate the uneconomic size of institutions at a high cost to society.[8]

A Preliminary Evaluation of HPEA
with Reference to Increasing the Number of Dentists

The Health Professions Education Act of 1963 was passed as a result of predictions of impending shortages of medical personnel in the United States. On the basis of these predictions a federal program was organized with the goal of subsidizing the "supply side" of the health manpower market. It was hoped that by 1975 the supply of personnel being produced by the nation's health training institutions should be sufficient to match the demands for personnel, so that the 1962 personnel-to-population ratios would be maintained. Today, nine years after the passage of the initial legislation, it would be worthwhile to attempt an evaluation of the effects it has had on the manpower supply — in particular, its effect on the supply of dentists.

In 1962 representatives of the American Dental Association testified before the House Interstate and Foreign Commerce Committee that there will be a shortage of 12,000 dentists by 1975. In order to have the 130,000 dentists "required" by 1975, the ADA reported, the number of dental school graduates would have to be expanded from 3,200 per year in 1962 to 6,200 graduates per year by 1975. This would require, the ADA said, increasing the capacity of existing dental schools so that they would graduate a total of 750 additional dentists per year by 1975, plus building 22 new schools, each to graduate approximately 100 students per year (see Table 4-7). In terms of yearly increments, this would mean an increase of 250 graduates per year.[9] Obviously, such a massive increase in capacity could only be achieved with federal assistance, which was soon forthcoming as part of the HPEA program.

Table 4-7. **Requirements for Increased Dental Graduates, American Dental Association, 1962**

Year	Number of Dental Schools	Enrollment	First-Year Students	Graduates
1962 (actual)[1]	47	13,513	3,605	3,207
1975 (forecast)	69[2]	27,900[3]	7,330[3]	6,200[2]

1. U.S. Department of Health Education, and Welfare, Public Health Service, Bureau of Health Professions Education and Manpower Training, *Health Manpower Source Book, Section 20: Manpower Supply and Educational Statistics for Selected Health Occupations,* Public Health Service Publication No. 263, Section 20. Updated as of March 3, 1971. U.S. Government Printing Office, Washington, D.C. (hereafter *Health Manpower Source Book*).

2. Summary Statement of the American Dental Association, in *Hearings,* January 23, 1962, p. 178.

3. Estimates based on normal numerical relationships between graduates, enrollment, and first-year places, over time.

In general, the HPEA program was designed to increase supply in two ways: by subsidizing students and by subsidizing dental schools. With regard to students, money was given to schools to distribute for scholarship purposes according to a formula that was related to class size multiplied by $1,500. Funds were also to be provided to schools ($35.7 million) to be used for student loans over the first three years of the program, with the maximum annual loan being $2,000.[10] With regard to subsidies to schools, federal funds were to be available for three general purposes: (1) construction of additional capacity, through the construction of new schools as well as by enlarging existing ones using federal matching funds; (2) grants to enable schools to improve the quality of their instruction, again through the use of matching funds; and (3) cost of education payments to assist the schools with the costs of educating the additional students who would be entering as a result of HPEA (since tuition only pays a portion of the total per student costs). The formula to be used for determining such cost of education subsidies was similar to that used for scholarships (but instead of $1,500, $1,000 was used).[11]

Data available for 1970-1971 and the intervening period since initiation of the program makes it possible to provide a preliminary evaluation of the effectiveness of the program as well as the bases upon which it was started.

An attempt at evaluating the HPEA act should examine the following areas:

1. The student loan and scholarship funds

2. Construction and improvement grants to new and existing schools

3. Cost of education subsidies to dental schools,

4. The accuracy of the original predictions and the basis upon which these support programs were made

The amounts of Federal funds provided for each of these objectives are shown in Table 4-8.

Table 4-8. Federal Funds for Dental Schools and Students Under the HPEA Grants Program, 1965-1971

	1965	1966	1967	1968	1969	1970	1971	Summary 1965-1971
School Construction	$19,237,774	$14,997,421	$35,861,608	$23,570,169	$24,186,339	$29,642,380	$27,097,781	$174,593,472
Number of Schools	8	5	9	6	3	9	7	
Institutional Support								
Formula Grants		$ 2,975,283	$ 8,440,653	$11,551,559	$17,935,630	$22,165,720	$24,964,441	$ 88,033,286
Number of Schools		49	52	50	51	51	52	
Project Grants		$ 2,975,283	$ 8,440,653	$ 8,862,500	$ 9,213,000	$ 9,204,031	$ 9,119,767	$ 47,815,234
Number of Schools								
				– $ 2,689,059	$ 8,722,630	$12,961,689	$15,844,674	$ 40,218,052
Number of Schools				11	26	35	36	
Student Support								
Scholarships	$ 2,870,963	$ 4,623,920	$ 7,940,200	$ 8,297,943	$ 9,131,979	$ 6,749,338	$ 8,475,924	$ 48,090,267
			$ 808,200	$ 1,475,826	$ 2,354,245	$ 3,164,945	$ 3,004,606	$ 10,807,822
Number of Schools			49	50	52	53	53	
Number of Students			799	1,869	3,135	4,092	4,036	
Average Scholarship			$ 1,012	$ 790	$ 751	$ 773	$ 774	
Loans	$ 2,870,963	$ 4,623,920	$ 7,132,000	$ 6,822,177	$ 6,777,734	$ 3,584,393	$ 5,471,318	$ 37,282,445
Number of Schools	46	46	46	47	50	52	52	
Number of Students	3,367	4,472	5,530	5,944	6,373	5,494	5,337	
Average Loan	$ 853	$ 1,034	$ 1,290	$ 1,148	$ 1,064	$ 652	$ 1,025	
							TOTAL	$310,717,025

Source: Division of Dental Health, National Institutes of Health, Department of Health, Education, and Welfare.

Note: Formula grants are grants to be used primarily for the support of teaching faculty and staff, acquiring equipment and supplies, and other costs associated with maintaining educational quality for enrollment increases and other expansion. Enligibility for these grants carries a statutory requirement of increased enrollment. Special project grants provide broad range assistance to schools for projects to expand enrollments, alleviate financial distress, or improve curriculum or methods of training. See U.S. Congress, *Senate Report of the Committee on Labor and Public Welfare on S. 934*, July 12, 1971, U.S. Government Printing Office, Washington, D.C., 1971, p. 10.

Student Loan and Scholarship Funds

If the objective of a loan and scholarship program is to increase the number of dentists, then such a program must attract the "marginal" student into dentistry. There are a certain number of students who will go into dentistry and are financially able to pay their own way. These students will enter dental school (if accepted) whether or not financial assistance is available. A second group of academically qualified college graduates may be financially able to enter dental school without financial aid, but may be uncertain as to whether or not they want to become dentists. Finally, a third group of academically qualified college students may wish to attend dental school but may not have the financial resources to do so. In order to increase the supply of dentists, financial inducements must be offered to the second and third groups to enter dental training.

The test of the effectiveness of the HPEA financial assistance program is this: which group received the bulk of the loan and scholarship money? If it was the first group, the funds only served to subsidize students who would have been willing to pay their own way. If it was the second and/or third group, then additional students will have been attracted to dentistry as a career who might not otherwise have become dentists; the financial assistance program will then have served to increase the supply of dentists.

Scholarship and loan programs may also have as their objective a change in the mix of students. If this were the case, then the measure of success of this objective would be similar to one which desires an increase in the number of students; namely, data indicating that students with different economic or minority group backgrounds are greater in number as a proportion of the total than previously.

The data required to evaluate the effectiveness of the student financial assistance aspects of the HPEA in the manner we would like are unavailable, as is noted below. It is unfortunate that the legislation did not require an evaluation to be made of how well the program goals were being achieved and whether fewer or greater amounts of money should be spent on each objective. It would be useful if, in the future, such data could be collected in the areas noted below, such that a more meaningful evaluation of the program could be undertaken.[12]

However, based on some preliminary data it is possible to draw some inferences regarding this aspect of the legislation. If the "marginal" student (i.e., one who is well qualified but would not select dentistry for reasons of either financial resources or other preferences) is to be attracted to dentistry, then we should be able to observe a change in the percentage of dental students who come from families of different economic backgrounds. The only data that is available on dental student-family income distribution are for 1963. These data are presented in Table 4-9.

Since no additional data have been collected as a result of the HPEA, one cannot say how this distribution has shifted over time. Although no data have been collected on the family income distribution of dental students beyond 1963, data are available for medical students for both 1963 and 1967. Since

Table 4-9. Dental Student Family Income Distribution, 1963

	Family Income			
	$0-4000	$4000-10,000	$10,000-15,000	$15,000+
Percent Dental Students	11.7[1]	56.3[2]	10.0[2]	22.0[1]
Percent Total Population[3]	27.2	52.8	14.5	5.4

1. U.S. Congress, Senate, *Hearings Before the Subcommittee on Labor and Public Welfare, on S. 595 and H.R. 3141,* September 8, 1965, Prepared Statement of the American Association of Dental Schools, U.S. Government Printing Office, Washington, D.C., 1965, p. 91.

2. Statement of Dr. Maynard K. Hine, President-Elect, Dean, School of Dentistry, Indiana University; Accompanied by Dr. A. Ray Baralt, Jr., Dean, School of Dentistry, University of Detroit; Dr. Reginald H. Sullens, Executive Secretary, American Association of Dental Schools; and Mr. Hal M. Christensen, Director of the Washington Office, American Dental Association, in *Hearings,* September 8, 1965, p. 75.

3. U.S. Bureau of the Census, *Statistical Abstract of the United States, 1965,* Washington, D.C., 1965, p. 341.

medical schools and medical students are also subsidized by the HPEA program, it may be useful to examine the medical student profile, as a proxy for the dental students, in an attempt to determine whether HPEA has been successful in bringing a greater proportion of lower income students into dentistry.

Table 4-10 compares the incomes of all families and of the families of medical students in 1963 and 1967. Based on this table, there has not been an increase in

Table 4-10. Family Incomes of All Families and of Families of Medical Students, 1963 and 1967

	1963		1967	
Family Income	Medical Students	All Families	Medical Students	All Families
TOTAL	100%	100%	100%	100%
Less than $5,000	15	36	9	25
$ 5,000 – 9,999	36	44	28	41
$10,000 – 14,999	20	15	22	22
$15,000 – 24,999	15	4	21	10
$25,000 or more	14	1	20	2

Source: Smith, Louis C. R., and Crocker, Anna R., *How Medical Students Finance Their Education,* U.S. Department of Health, Education, and Welfare, Public Health Service Publication No. 1336-1, U.S. Government Printing Office, Washington, 1970, p. 8.

the proportion of medical students from families with lower incomes. There has, however, been a shift in the distribution of family incomes between 1963 and

1967, but the relative position of family incomes of medical students has not appeared to have changed. If one assumes that the HPEA program has been similarly administered with dental students, then it would have been equally unsuccessful in changing the proportion of dental students coming from lower income families. This comparison is based on 1967 data, which was only the third year in which the HPEA program was even partially in operation. A more complete evaluation must wait for later data, if it becomes available.

The percentage of dental students receiving financial assistance was much greater in 1970 than in 1962, which was before the HPEA was in existence (see Table 4-11). However, tuition costs increased far more rapidly from 1962 to 1970 than did the average value of the award. Surprisingly, though, the percentage of students needing assistance went down over that period, from 60 percent to 40 percent. With the large increases in tuition costs relative to income, one would expect that many more students would require financial assistance, unless they came from families with sufficient family resources to assist them, or received additional funds from working or from loans that are not part of the HPEA program. Since such data are unavailable it is not possible to substantiate any of these hypotheses.

Another consideration in attempting to evaluate the impact of the student financial assistance portion of the HPEA is whether there has been a reduction in

Table 4-11. Student Financial Assistance and Tuition Costs, 1962 and 1970

Year	Average Yearly Tuition Cost	Total 4-Year Expense	Financial Assistance		Average Annual Value of Award	
			Percent Needing	Percent Receiving	Loan	Scholarship
1962	$ 800[1]	$15,000[1]	60[2]	13[2]	$627[2]	$480[2]
1970	$2000[3]	$22,500[4]	40[5]	33[5]	$666[5]	$774[5]

1. Summary Statement of the American Dental Association, in *Hearings,* January 23, 1962, Op Cit., p. 179.

2. Supplementary Statement of the American Dental Association, in *Hearings,* January 23, 1962, Op Cit., p. 182.

3. U.S. Congress, Senate, *Hearings Before the Subcommittee on Health of the Committee on Labor and Public Welfare,* September 2 and 4, 1970. Prepared Statement of David A. Bensinger, D.D.S., Assistant Dean, Washington University, School of Dentistry, St. Louis, Mo. U.S. Government Printing Office, Washington, D.C., 1970, p. 87.

4. U.S. Congress, House of Representatives, *Hearings Before the Subcommittee on Public Health and Environment of the Committee on Interstate and Foreign Commerce, on H.R. 703, 4171, 4155, 5614, 5767, 7765, 4145, 4156, 4718, 7707, 7736,* April 2, 3, 20, 21, 22, 23, 27, 28, 29, 1971. Statement of Dr. James W. Bowden, Dean, University of North Carolina School of Dentistry, in behalf of the American Dental Association and American Association of Dental Schools; Accompanied by Dr. Richard R. Mosbaugh, Chairman, Council on Legislation, ADA, and Hal M. Christensen, Director, Washington Office, ADA, U.S. Government Printing Office, Washington, D.C., 1971, p. 717.

5. Ibid., p. 711.

the number of student dropouts as a result of additional financial assistance. Again, the data are not sufficient to permit us to draw any conclusions in this regard. As shown in Table 4-12, from 1964-1966 the percentage of dental students failing to complete their education has been greater than 11 percent.

Table 4-12. Students Failing to Complete Their Dental Education

Year of Graduation	1st-Year Students, 4 Years Earlier	Number of Graduates	"Dropouts"	"Dropouts" as Percent of Original Class Size
1970	3,942	3,500	442	11.2
1969	3,806	3,433	373	9.8
1968	3,836	3,457	379	9.9
1967	3,770	3,360	410	10.9
1966	3,680	3,198	482	13.1
1965	3,605	3,181	424	11.8
1964	3,616	3,213	403	11.1
TOTAL	26,255	23,342	2,913	11.1

Source: U.S. Department of Health, Education, and Welfare, Public Health Service, National Institutes of Health, Bureau of Health Manpower Education, *Health Manpower Source Book: Manpower Supply and Educational Statistics,* Updated as of March, 1971. P.H.S. Publication No. 263 – Section 20, p. 6.

Then for 1967-1969 this percentage declined; but for the most recent year for which data are available (1970) it has risen again to over 11 percent.

The objective of the HPEA is presumably to increase the number of dentists in the population rather than the number of dentists going into a specialty practice. It would therefore be useful to determine, for administrative purposes, whether loans and other financial assistance are provided to students who become specialists. Since dental specialists require additional training, the availability of funds to such students might provide them with an incentive to undertake such additional training. Since dental specialists are limited to practice only in their specialty, the supply of nonspecialists will increase more rapidly if no inducements were provided for specialty training. (Such a policy might suggest, in addition to denying financial assistance for specialty training, the repayment of all previous financial assistance for persons undertaking specialty training.)

As shown earlier, the number of specialists has been increasing as a percentage of total dentists. There are a number of possible reasons for this, such as a higher rate of return; however, the administration of student financial assistance should be in accordance with the presumed goal of increasing the number of dentists rather than the number of specialists. It would thus appear that the objectives underlying the student financial assistance aspect of the HPEA program are not altogether explicit. If it is desired to change the mix of the student body then it is not clear why funds for students are provided to dental schools on criteria other than the number of needy students, e.g., providing the schools with a choice of using as a basis for support the size of their student body rather than the number of low income students. Further, if the objective was to induce graduates to locate in low income areas why provide funds only to the needy (regardless of where they may locate)?

One final comment is in order with regard to the logic of the student assistance aspects of the HPEA. Since it appears that the major constraint to the production of more graduates is the number of dental school spaces — i.e., there are always more applicants than acceptances — and the number of applicants has been increasing, providing financial assistance to students will not increase the number of entrants but will instead only increase the pool of applicants from which schools can select their specified number of entrants. The rate of return to a dental education is already greater than a "normal" rate of return to such an education. Therefore, subsidizing students will serve to increase the rate of return to those receiving such financial assistance. As long as there are constraints on the number of spaces, subsidizing students will not increase the number of graduates but will enable those spaces to be filled from a larger choice of students, either on the basis of background (e.g., financial or cultural) or on the basis of grades.

Since it is the dental schools that determine the number of dental students, it is with respect to dental school subsidies and their additional output of graduates that the entire effectiveness of the HPEA program is determined. This is the next aspect of the legislation to be examined.

Construction and Improvement Grants
to New and Existing Schools

The amount of both construction and improvement grants (to provide for upgrading and improvement in the quality of the institution) provided under HPEA are summarized in Table 4-13. Total construction and project grants between 1964 and 1971 amounted to over $173 million. Annual construction expenditures alone averaged $21,000,000 a year and over a seven-year period created 1,123 new first-year places; 396 were created by building six new schools and 727 were created through expansion of 29 existing schools. Additionally, another $100 million in federal funds for construction projects had been approved by March 1971, to result in 443 more new first-year places.[13] Institutional support for improvement has been increasing from less than $3 million a year in 1966 to almost $25 million by 1971 (cf. Table 4-9). Planned expenditures for such institutional support are expected to sharply increase in amount from 1971 to 1975.[14]

An important question with respect to the effect of such federal matching funds for creating new spaces is how much additional capacity was created as a result of such funds which would not otherwise have been constructed. Since federal funds were available, construction that would have been undertaken

Table 4-13. Health Professions Educational Assistance Construction Program Summary, Fiscal Years 1965-1971 (As of May 26, 1971)

	Number of Schools	New First-Year Places	Federal Share	Total Cost	Federal Share per Place	Total Cost per Place
Dental, Total	35	1123	$173,255,166	$345,577,920	$154,252.15	$307,727.44
New Schools	6	396	43,610,192	68,525,945	110,126.75	173,045.32
Existing Schools	29	727	129,014,974	277,051,975	177,462.14	381,089.37

Source: U.S. Congress, Senate, *Report of the Committee on Labor and Public Welfare, on S. 934*, July 12, 1971, U.S. Government Printing Office, Washington, D.C., 1971, p. 8.

Note: The figure given above for total number of schools receiving construction aid is less than the sum of the yearly recipients of aid as given in Table 3. This is probably due to a "double counting" of schools in the yearly totals of Table 3, that is, a school may have received funds in more than one year, and thus may be represented in the total for more than one year.

without the HPEA was now presumably subsidized by the HPEA. It would be important, in evaluating the construction aspect of the program, to determine what percentage of new places was created only because of the availability of federal matching funds.

This, of course, is difficult to determine. Our only indication as to how many places were created solely because of the availability of federal funds is the statement of dental school plans. For example, in 1962 the ADA representatives, in testimony before Congressional committees, said that dental schools had expansion plans to result in a total of 354 new first-year places; however with federal aid, those plans would be increased so that 725 new places would be created.[15] In Chapter 5 an attempt is made using an econometric model of the dental care sector to simulate the effect on dental prices, visits, and expenditures of the construction portion of the HPEA. This simulation is then compared to another simulation that assumes no HPEA (therefore less construction funds, hence fewer dentists).

There are some interesting aspects on the allocation of these funds between existing and new schools. First, the vast majority of these funds went to existing schools. Second, that each additional first-year place created by constructing new schools was built at a cost of $110,126 of federal funds. Each additional space created by expanding existing schools was built at a cost of $177,462 of federal funds. (The total cost per space, including federal and matching funds, was $173,045 and $381,089, respectively; see Table 4-13.) One would expect that it would be much less expensive to expand existing schools than to create new schools. It therefore appears that the large amount of funds per space in existing schools also served to "upgrade" these schools rather than just create increments to the supply of dentists.

As for the use of the special and basic improvement grant funds, it also appears that they may not have been entirely spent on the purpose for which they were granted. One report stated, "Much of the functioning under special project grant authority has been to alleviate financial distress rather than to assure institutional and program innovation, such as curriculum reform."[16]

One aspect of the construction program that is useful to note is the position of the new schools receiving federal funds on the cost curve for producing new students. For example, the six new schools created between 1965 and 1971 averaged only 66 new first-year places per school, as opposed to the original ADA goal of building new schools capable of graduating 100 students per year. Hopefully, schools receiving federal funds would increase their class sizes, hence decreasing their per unit costs.

Cost of Education Subsidies to Dental Schools

In 1962, dental student tuition represented approximately 30 percent of the cost of education.[17] The HPEA therefore provided for "cost of education" payments to schools to assist them in handling the additional students enrolling as a result of the federally financed school capacity and student assitance programs. However, it appears that such "cost of education" subsidies went to schools regardless of how much they increased their enrollment. A flat $1,000 payment to the school per student would appear to be more favorable to the larger schools whose per unit costs are lower; such a subsidy program would be desirable if it provided an incentive to schools with higher per unit costs to increase their enrollment and thus lower their unit costs.

But what if subsidies were given on the basis of the per student cost for the largest enrollment category of schools, thus tending to force all schools to operate at enrollments which lead to lower average costs per student? What savings in the program could then have been realized? If the purpose of the cost of education subsidy was to cause an increase in enrollment for the above purpose, then the method used in the HPEA for allocating such subsidies did not achieve this. Other than subsidizing the schools it is not clear what the objectives were of such a subsidy. It was not tied to specific enrollment increases and did not require schools to take advantage of economies of scale (in the sense of serving as an incentive), since other funds such as project grants for improvement were available from the HPEA.[18]

Accuracy of Original Forecasts

In the above discussion of HPEA, various parts of the legislation were considered in order to determine whether and how much of an effect each of the funding programs had on increasing dental manpower in accordance with the goals proposed in 1962. In this section we wish to examine the original goals underlying the HPEA.

The basis for Federal funding was to maintain the current dentist-population ratio through 1975. One might therefore ask:

1. How accurate were the population and dentist supply estimates, which were the underpinnings of the entire program?
2. Were the funds requested sufficient to achieve the goals established?
3. Was the maintenance of a dentist-population ratio the proper basis for undertaking such a large program?

In 1962 the American Dental Association forecast for 1975 a population of 230 million people. In 1971 the Division of Dental Health, Department of Health, Education, and Welfare, produced a 1975 population forecast of only 217,550,000.[19] In order to maintain the 1962 dentist-population ratio of 1,945:1 only 114,500 dentists would be needed, according to this latter population estimate, not the 130,000 originally believed necessary.

In making its appeal to Congress for federal aid to dental education the American Dental Association predicted that a dentist supply of 118,000 would be forthcoming without any assistance; federal support was required in order to eliminate the expected 12,000 "deficit" and bring the supply into equality with the "needs" for 130,000 dentists. The desired legislation was passed and federal aid initiated which, if a more accurate population estimate had been available at that time, would have been unnecessary, if the goal was to maintain the 1962 dentist-population ratio.

Also, according to the 1971 revised estimates by HEW, the forthcoming dentist supply in 1975 is more likely to be 111,400 *with* the federal assistance program, which is 6,600 less than was estimated by the ADA in 1962 without any federal assistance.

The purpose of this discussion is not to use hindsight to criticize early forecasts of population and dentist supply. It is difficult to make accurate forecasts thirteen years ahead. However, it seems that when a federal program is requested, costing several hundred million dollars, more sophisticated techniques should be used for estimating future number of dentists and population, and the estimates should be continually updated. Further, when such estimates can be subject to such wide error, flexibility should be built into the program so that it can be revised as the need arises.

In 1962 Dr. Raymond Nagle, representing the American Dental Association, testified as to the program requirements which would generate 250 new dental graduates per year at a cost of *$350 million* in total by 1975. The number of dental graduates in 1962 was 3,207. Therefore 250 additional dentists per year for twelve years would, by 1975, result in almost doubling the yearly number of graduates to approximately 6,200 per year.

Proposed Program

1. Rehabilitate existing schools which have outmoded/outworn buildings and equipment, such that there will be no reduction in their enrollment.

2. Most of the existing (1962) 47 schools must add the facilities needed to graduate 750 more dentists in the next ten years, an average of 16 additional dentists per school by 1972.

3. At least 22 new schools, each to graduate about 100 dentists per year, must be constructed at a cost of approximately $6 million per school.

4. For scholarship/loan and cost of education aid, a program was requested in the form of the formulas described earlier.[21]

Thus, under the proposed program, the majority of the additional graduates (2,200 per year) were to come from new schools. Later data show that these financial requests have been substantially met by the Health Professions Educational Assistance program. For example, $150 million in federal construction funds were requested for the period 1962-1972; as of May 26, 1971, $173,225,166 had already been supplied. Non-federal matching construction funds also exceeded expectations. Institutional support for the years 1966-1971 totaled $88,033,286. Student support aid, totaling $57,619,716 for the years 1965-1972, also substantially met originally stated needs.

The goals which were to be met by such a large federal expenditure, however, were not achieved. Twenty-two new dental schools were desired by 1975; in

1971, with only four years to go, only six new schools had been constructed (two of which had been planned prior to the HPEA), and a net of only four more will be ready by 1975. (This indicates that the existing schools received a much larger share of the projected financial support than was originally proposed.) Annual dental school graduates were to number 6,200 in 1975; thus far, graduates have increased from 3,233 in 1963 to only 3,500 in 1970, and are currently expected to reach only 4,270 by 1975. The goal of 130,000 dentists will be missed by a shortfall of almost 20,000.[22]

The HPEA program has resulted in an increase in the supply of dentists over what it would otherwise have been. However, could the increase in supply have been greater had the funds been provided to existing schools with more inducements to increase their enrollment?

There has been a great disparity between predictions and that which is realized, and between program goals and program achievements. Such program funds could presumably have been spent in other areas, and if trade-offs are to be made between alternative uses of such scarce funds, better information on which to base these comparisons is clearly needed.

Maintenance of a Dentist-Population Ratio as a
Basis for Federal Support

A Federal program, once started, begins to have a life of its own. A constituency is developed and regardless of whether its goals are being attained, or even whether other programs have more pressing needs, it becomes difficult to change the direction of that program. It is important therefore to analyze the basic premises underlying new programs, since that is the time at which they are most likely to be changed. Although it is too late to do this in regard to the HPEA, we might still perform the exercise if for no other purpose than to hope that data on accomplishments and a clearer specification of future goals would be forthcoming.

Dentists are only one factor, albeit the most important one, in the production of dental services. Therefore, if there was concern that there should be an adequate supply of dental care available in 1975, then the emphasis should perhaps have been based not on maintaining a dentist-population ratio but on a dental care services (or visit)-to-population ratio. The emphasis on this latter ratio might have resulted in different estimates of the magnitude and type of federal support required to maintain such a ratio. Analogously, few people would be in favor of maintaining the ratio of farmers per thousand population that existed at any time in the past. Farmers are a prime factor in the production of food; however, any program based on the maintenance of a given farmer-population ratio would have been seriously in error, if other factors contributing to increased productivity were not also considered.

One might even question maintaining a fixed ratio of any service to population. For one thing, if demand for that service increases, then the desired ratio of that service to the population will be too small. To be able to forecast the future dental population ratio, therefore, one would have to estimate the demand for dental care, the likely portion of that care that will be provided by dentists, and then, the future population, and the forthcoming supplies of dentists and auxiliaries. It makes one wonder why the dentist-population ratio should be subsidized in the first place. (This question is discussed more completely in Chapter 6 on financing dental care.) However, for the remainder of this discussion it is assumed that the objective of the HPEA was to insure a certain minimum supply of dental care by 1971. The question then is, what would have been the likely supply of dental care available in relation to the population *without* the HPEA federal assistance, when viewed at the time of the HPEA hearings?

When one rereads the testimony of various persons and organizations at the time the HPEA was proposed, it is easy to become confused as to which population-dentist-ratio was to be maintained to 1975. For example, Dr. Raymond Nagle, representing the American Dental Association, testified during the hearings in January 1962 that, given an expected 1975 population of 230 million, 130,000 *active* dentists would be necessary to maintain the 1961 population-dentist ratio of 1900:1 (185,000,000:95,000 practicing dentists). The 1975 supply of dentists, given no federal assistance, was forecast as 118,000.

In actuality, though, a ratio of 185 million people to 95,000 dentists is 1,947:1, not 1,900:1. Further, a ratio of 230 million people to 118,000 dentists would be 1,950:1; thus, in 1975 the forecast supply of dentists, with no federal assistance, would have been almost sufficient to maintain the actual 1961 population–dentist ratio of 1,947:1.

Since the 1975 population-dentist ratio, using the ADA's forecast of population and dentist supply in 1975, would be approximately the same as that prevailed in 1961, it is not clear what ratio the ADA intended to maintain with these 130,000 dentists. Where then did the "shortage" of 12,000 dentists come from? Apparently the "needed" 130,000 dentists in 1975 is not based on maintaining the 1961 dentist-population ratio but rather the 1958 ratio. If one calculates the population-dentist ratio in 1975 with 230 million people and 130,000 dentists then it is 1,767:1 − much lower than the 1961 ratio. When Dr. Nagle testified that "several expert groups" said 130,000 dentists was the number that would be necessary to maintain to 1975 the level of dental services available "today" (1962), we examined the reports of some of those expert groups.[23]

Complicating further the investigation of the "ratio" to be maintained was the use of "active" and "practicing" dentists versus total dentists. As discussed earlier, there are two different series on dentists, the ADA series refers to total dentists and the HEW series has both total and active dentists.

We examined the Bane report, it being the best known of the five studies mentioned by Dr. Nagle. The Bane report stated that at the "current" (1958) levels of dental school output, the *total* dentist supply would reach 118,000 in

1975. To meet the needs associated with population growth (i.e., to maintain the 1958 population-dentist ratio) would require a *total* of 134,000 dentists. These figures for *total* dentists expected and needed in 1975 (118,000 and 134,000) are approximately those presented by Dr. Nagle as the figures for *active* dentists expected and needed in 1975.

Thus it appears that Dr. Nagle in his Congressional testimony accidently talked in terms of active practicing dentists in 1961 when the data on which he was basing his presentation was in terms of total dentists, and the ratio to be maintained was not of 1961 but rather of 1958. Since "total" dentists are composed of "active practicing" dentists plus retired dentists, a ratio of population to total dentists will require fewer active dentists than a ratio of (the same) population to active dentists. The error of trying to maintain the 1958 population − total dentist ratio as a population − active dentist ratio in 1975 therefore gives the impression that more dentists are required.

This discussion had dealt only with an understanding of the figures used by the American Dental Association in testifying on behalf of Federal aid to dental education. We have talked in terms of "dentists required to maintain population-dentist ratios," as a measure of sustaining a level of dental services.

There is however another way of examining the likely dental supply population ratio, and that is to look at the expected visit-population rate that existed in 1961 (or 1958 for that matter) and what visit-population rate would have been expected in 1975. In 1961 the visit rate was 1.6546 visits per person (in 1958 it was 1.7711 visits per person.) The method used to calculate the visit-population rate for different time periods was to use the mean visits per dentist with different numbers of auxiliaries and multiply these by the number of dentists using each such dental auxiliary combination in a particular period. Summing overall dentists would then provide an estimate of the total number of visits, which, when divided by the population, would equal the visit-population rate.

Using *Survey of Dental Practice* data on mean patient visits per dentist, *Statistical Abstract* data on total resident population, and *Distribution of Dentist* data on dentist supply, it is possible to calculate visit-population rate of 1.7201 for 1958 and 1.7193 for 1961. These differ from the rate for those years presented in the section on the ADA's testimony in favor of HPEA. The difference between these two sets of figures is due to the use of different figures for the number of dentists. Whereas the 1.7201 and 1.7193 rates were derived using the ADA's published dentist figures, the visit rates of 1.6546 and 1.7711 used the dentist figures given by the ADA in their testimony. These latter dentist figures differ from the *Distribution of Dentists* numbers; in fact they turn out to be similar to HEW's published figures. The same population and visit per dentist data was used in calculating both sets of rates, hence the two sets differ only due to the different dentist supply totals used. To be consistent therefore, we have calculated the visit-population rate using the same number of total dentists as was used in the testimony.

If we accept the 1975 forecast of population and dentists made in 1962 by the ADA then the visit *rate* in 1975 would have been *1.6531* per person without the HPEA program. This is based on the assumption that there will be the same use of auxiliaries by dentists in 1975 as in 1961 and also the same productivity of each dentist-auxiliary mix in 1975 as in 1961. The projected (in 1962) 1975 dentist supply without the HPEA program would therefore have been sufficient to supply the projected 1975 population with almost exactly the same number of visits per person as were provided in 1961 (1.6564 in 1961; 1.6530 in 1975). Given increased use of auxiliaries by dentists in 1975 (i.e., more auxiliaries employed per dentist) and increased productivity by the dentist-auxiliary "team," the projected supply of dentists could provide even *more* visits per capita in 1975 than was supplied in 1961.

This means that, measured on a visit basis, service in 1975 would have been at least identically available, and probably even more available than it was in 1961. For example, given a continuation of the increases in dentist productivity, which have been estimated by several investigators, the projected (in 1962) dentist supply in 1975 would be able to provide even *more* visits per capita than were available in 1961 or 1958. If dental productivity (the number of visits per dentist) were to increase by 1 percent per year starting in 1962 then the visit rate would be 1.8813 per person in 1975. A 1 percent increase in dental productivity has been estimated as the increase in productivity attributable solely to technical change. A 3 percent increase in dental productivity has been estimated as the rate of increase that actually prevailed during 1950-1970. If the 3 percent increase in productivity were to prevail for the period 1962-1975 then the visit rate in 1975 would be 2.4277.

For the purpose of comparison with the forecasts of dental services made in 1958 and in 1962, the 1970 visit-population rate was calculated, based on 1970 *Survey of Dental Practice* visit data. The increase in the 1970 visit-population rate was in part a result of an increase in average dental productivity, through greater use of auxiliaries and from greater productivity of each dentist-auxiliary combination. Note that (1) the dentist supply grew absolutely between 1962 and 1970; (2) an increase in the mean visits per-dentist occured between 1961 and 1970 (3119 to 3565); and (3) dentists were employing more auxiliaries in 1970 than in 1961. The result was a 31.5 percent increase in total visits between 1962 and 1970; with population increasing only by 10.1 percent over this period, the visit-population rate increased from 1.6546 to 1.8128. This increase of 31.5 percent in "provision of dental services" despite an increase of only 7.2 percent in the input of dentists illustrates the possibilities for increasing the provision of services by increasing the other (presumably cheaper and shorter in time to produce) inputs — equipment and auxiliary personnel. It also illustrates the fallacy of viewing the problem of providing dental services as solely one of providing dentists.

In summary therefore, the ADA's forecast in 1962 of population and dental supply for 1975 would have been sufficient, in the absence of federal legislation, to maintain either the 1958 or 1961 visit-population rate. If a continuation of the increases in dental productivity, as estimated by several investigators, were incorporated into the forecast 1975 dental supply, it would have indicated that the visit-population rate would have exceeded any previous estimates. Measured in terms of visits, therefore (which is really a better measure of service than just the number of dentists), forecasts of dental service would have predicted it to be at least as available, and probably more available, in 1975 than in 1958 or 1961 even without any federal aid to dental education.

Concluding Comments on HPEA

This section has attempted an analysis of that part of the HPEA program related to dentistry. It has been preliminary and incomplete, since sufficient data are not currently available to undertake a more substantive analysis. Perhaps the most obvious conclusion from such an analysis is that a program costing several hundred million dollars should be given a proper evaluation — one that would include an examination of its objectives and whether there are alternatives to achieving these objectives which can be less expensive. An evaluation of this program should also relate the results of such a program to the rest of the dental sector so as to determine whether there are perhaps other goals with respect to dental care that will have a higher return per federal dollar spent on them. The HPEA should not be evaluated in isolation from other federal programs in dental health nor without respect to these other objectives. Unless such a broader examination of the HPEA is undertaken it will not be possible to determine the trade-offs between manpower and other programs for improving the oral health status of the population.

With regard to the more limited objective of increasing dental manpower, it would appear that analyses of the effects of the various financial assistance programs should also be undertaken, in addition to the development of more accurate population forecasts and the determinants of the long-run supply of dentists. The prime beneficiaries of the HPEA appear to have been the students receiving financial assistance and the dental schools themselves.

The existing dental schools have received most of the available federal funds for construction, improvement, special purposes, and for student support. They have been able to upgrade their facilities and faculties, select from a larger pool of applicants, and receive relief from their financial difficulties. The "quid pro quo" that has been extracted from these schools for receiving these benefits has been, to date, small increases in enrollment and insufficient data to determine whether there has been a change in the mix of their student body, whether there has been curriculum reform for reducing the time required to produce an additional dentist, or whether there have been any changes in the wide variations among schools in costs to produce dentists. Since the goals of the institutions receiving the funds may not be coincident with the stated objectives underlying the provision of federal funds, the achievement of such objectives should be continually monitored. Any exemptions by the schools from meeting such goals should be carefully scrutinized — e.g., the practice of requesting an exemption from increasing enrollment once a school has received capitation grants.

There has been an increase in the number of dentists, which was greater than what would have occurred without the HPEA. However, could an increase in supply of dental care have been achieved at lower cost if dental school financial assitance had been based on greater enrollment increases and on curriculum changes in order to produce dental manpower in shorter periods of time? Further, if the increased supply of dentists as a result of the HPEA were to benefit those who need it most, should perhaps a greater portion of the HPEA have been oriented to producing dental care and dentists in areas with the greatest needs for dental care?[25]

Government Financing of Dental and Auxiliary Education

Educational facilities in the dental sector are important determinants of the inputs into the provision of dental care — dental schools being more significant since on-the-job training cannot be substituted for formal education as has been the case with dental auxiliaries. Therefore, an examination was made of the supply and demand for educational training of dentists and dental auxiliaries in order to determine (1) whether these markets are performing efficiently, and (2) how effective the government funds are that are spent in subsidizing these markets.

As regards the efficient performance of this industry, it appears that there are sufficient demands for dental and dental auxiliary training, that the supply responds to these demands in the areas of dental auxiliary training, but that dental schools have been unresponsive. It also appears that the cost of producing dental students varies greatly, not just because of quality differences but because many schools do not operate at an efficient size. It would appear, therefore, that the lack of supply response by dental schools has been an important limiting factor in increasing the supply of dentists. The effect of such restrictions is to increase the price of dental care to consumers and to restrict its availability. The proponents of such policies would undoubtedly claim that "quality" is maintained, but this would be difficult to prove and comes at a cost to the public of higher prices and less available care.

As regards the role of government financing of the demanders and the suppliers of education in these markets, it would appear that subsidizing dental students would merely increase their rate of return while enabling the schools to be more selective. Subsidies to the dental schools have, to date, resulted in only small increases in the output of dentists. The supply of training facilities for dental auxiliaries appears to respond well to the increased demand for such training. Since this market appears to be functioning efficiently, it is not clear why these markets must be subsidized at all. If these markets are functioning efficiently, then the only reason for subsidizing them would be to increase their output even more and bring about a slightly lower price of the final product, namely, dental care. The subsidization of any part of the dental education sector would presumably have the same goal, namely, an increased number of graduates, greater availability of dental care (as a result of increased supply) and a lower price of dental care. If a subsidy is given to this sector, then it should be directed to the "marginal" student and not be for subsidization of the school itself. With an increase in demand for such training by students, such schools should respond to these demands as they have in the past. A subsidy to the school would not necessarily result in an increased enrollment unless the size of the subsidy were directly tied to such enrollment increases.

Unless there are other reasons for subsidizing such markets, then there are alternative financing mechanisms for achieving lower prices and an increase in quantity of dental care to desired population groups. One such alternative would be the financing of the demand for dental care, perhaps for specific population groups. However, even with increased demand for dental care, and increased demand by students for dental education, if the dental schools do not respond, then the price of dental care will rise rapidly, as will dental incomes.

The financing of dental schools might be viewed as a means of increasing the supply of dentists in a very nonresponsive market. If this were in fact the purpose, namely an increase in the supply of dentists, then it is possible to specify alternatives for increasing the dentist supply. The most obvious (and probably least acceptable to the dental profession) is to award a dental license on the basis of a uniform examination rather than have the additional prerequisite of having attended an accredited school for a minimum number of years.

Every professional organization attempts to increase the "quality" of its membership. This usually consists of increasing the training time required to be a professional, formal licensing requirements to enter the profession, as well as limitations on which tasks can be performed by different professions. Whatever the intentions underlying such proposals, the effect is usually the same — it increases the incomes of those currently in the profession by effectively reducing the supply from what it would have been without such restrictions. Given this economic behavior of professional organizations, one could predict that training requirements for becoming a dentist will not be decreased but in fact increased in the years ahead — as has been the case in medicine; and that the education requirements for becoming a dental auxiliary will also be increased and other restrictions imposed, if their professional organizations have the political ability to carry this out.

Appendix 4A.
An Empirical Analysis of
Economies of Scale in
Dental Education

An attempt was made to empirically determine the extent of economies of scale in dental schools. These results should be considered tentative since there are a number of data problems in such an analysis and also the empirical analyses were not able to explain a large amount of the variation in average cost per student among dental schools.

Separate analyses were undertaken for both private and public dental schools. The data for these analyses were for the years 1968-1969 and 1969-1970 collected by the Council on Dental Education, American Dental Association. For each type of school two sets of regressions were estimated; the first set of regressions estimated average cost per student (defined as the total cost of regular dental school programs divided by total enrollment) as a function of students, students-squared, and students-cubed. Although we received significant results for private schools, the results of these analyses with respect to public dental schools were all statistically insignificant. The second set of regressions attempted to adjust the average cost per student for differences in dental school salaries.

Because of the lack of data on number of faculty and their salaries in each school, the adjustment procedure was indirect; it consisted of multiplying each school's enrollment by the difference between the mean net salary of all dentists in the United States and the mean net salary of all dentists in the specific state; subtracting this product from the school's total cost, and dividing this figure by the enrollment to obtain the school's adjusted average cost.

All regressions contained dummy variables for the 1968-1969 and 1969-1970 school years, and are summarized in Table 4A.

Public Dental Schools. Only the first order term in the public school equation was statistically significant. The interpretation of this finding is that average cost per student in public dental schools declines over the range of observations for which we have data. This relationship is shown in Figure 4-2. Since the percent of the variation in average cost per student that was accounted for by the equation was only .25, a majority of the interschool variation in average cost per student is unexplained. There are several possible reasons for this finding that might also affect the estimate of average cost per student with different class sizes: One reason is that there is probably a large variation in the cost accounting methods used among schools. Another is that the "regular dental school program" may involve different "product mixes," for example GPs versus specialists, D.D.S. degree students versus graduate students, etc., for different schools. A further reason is the allocation problem between research and

135

Table 4A. Regression Results of Costs of Dental School Education

Regression No.	School Category	Dependent Variable	Coefficient of Independent Variable (T-Statistic)							
			Students	Students Squared	Students Cubed	Y1968	Y1969	R Squared	S.E.	N
1	Private	Average Cost	− 93.90 (−4.86)[1]	.2319 (4.07)[1]	−.00018 (−3.59)[1]	16,665 (8.51)[1]	17,355 (8.87)[1]	.52	1684.79	46
2	Private	Adjusted Average Cost	−167.11 (−6.58)[1]	.4490 (5.99)[1]	−.00036 (−5.49)[1]	23,562 (9.16)[1]	24,182 (9.41)[1]	.55	2214.69	46
3	Public	Adjusted Average Cost	− 36.75 (−1.83)[2]	.0320 (1.11)	—	16,572 (5.02)[1]	17,629 (5.29)[1]	.27	2928.47	48
4	Public	Adjusted Average Cost	− 14.83 (−3.75)[1]	—	—	13,225 (9.81)[1]	14,266 (10.22)[1]	.25	2936.08	48

1. Significant at .005 level
2. Significant at .05 level

Sources: Mean salaries of dentists, by state: American Dental Association, *1971 Survey of Dental Practice.* Enrollments and total costs, by school: American Dental Association, Council on Dental Education Correspondence with James A. Mastro, Project Director, Annual Report on Dental Education.

teaching in those schools, particularly the larger ones where there are more research grants, which grants might have the effect of subsidizing instructional costs. A last possible explanation for the per unit cost differences between schools is that there may be both quality and efficiency differences between schools that are difficult to measure and thus have not been accounted for.

Private Dental Schools. The empirical analyses of private dental schools was somewhat surprising. In the regressions using unadjusted average costs, there are two relative minimum cost areas; the first occurs at an enrollment of 327 students and then average costs rise until a class size of 532 students is reached and then declines again. When adjusted average cost is used in the regressions, the minimum occurs at 282 students, rises until 549 students and then declines.

Figure 4-2. Adjusted Average Cost per Student in Public Dental Schools, 1968, 1969

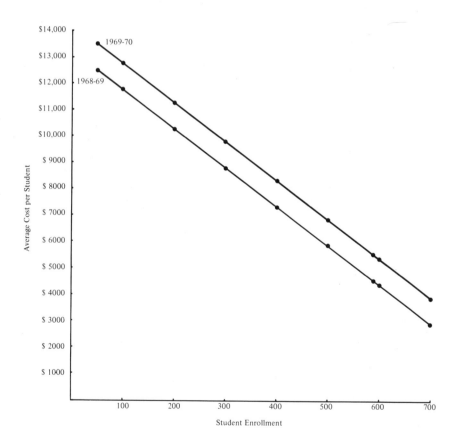

This relationship is shown in Figure 4-3. The percent of the variation accounted for in interschool average costs is .55. However, we are unable to explain the cause of this double minimum cost curve. One possible explanation is that as the schools increase in size beyond the area of the first minimum point, they begin to produce a different type of product (in terms of the types of instructional programs and amount of research efforts), and research grants begin to subsidize a greater percent of the instructional expenses.

Figure 4-3. Adjusted Average Cost per Student in Private Dental Schools, 1968, 1969

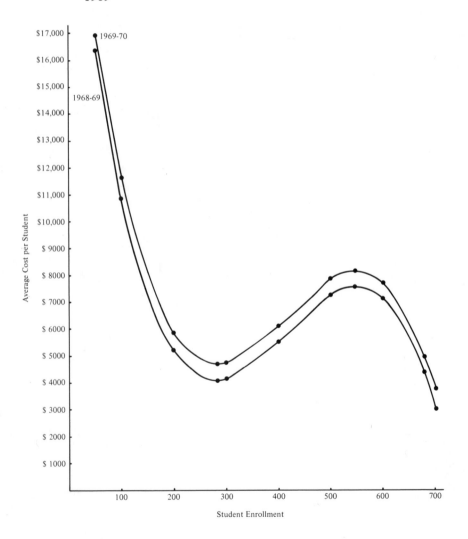

Even from these preliminary findings, it appears that economies of scale exist with regard to dental schools. However, the exact form of the cost functions remain somewhat unspecified and unexplained, particularly the large scatter of observations for public dental schools and the double-minimum character of the private school function.

Further research is called for in this area if the optimal operating point for dental schools is to be determined. Determination of this point would prove very valuable, for it would result in the building and/or expanding of facilities to the most efficient size. More standardized cost accounting procedures and record keeping, together with better measures of the costs of each type of dental school "product" are required if we are to be able to estimate the differences in costs that are a result of economies of scale, differences in quality and differences in the efficiency of the operation.[1]

5

An Econometric Model for
Forecasting and Policy
Evaluation in the
Dental Sector

The Uses of an Econometric Model

The traditional approach used in the dental sector for forecasting and planning is to view each segment separately. Forecasts are made of dental utilization, of the likely supply of dentists, and policies are proposed that will have the effect of changing some aspect of either supply or demand. No attempt is made to incorporate the effect of a change in one area on other areas that are likely to be affected.

In reality, however, the supply of dental services and the demand for these services are not determined separately; they are determined through interaction in a "dental care market." Therefore, if the effects of policies and of factors affecting demand and supply are to be anticipated correctly, the seemingly separate aspects of the dental sector must be considered together. The primary value of an econometric model is that it enables us to view the dental sector as an interrelated system. Once such a market system has been specified and estimated, and forecasts made of the factors affecting demand and supply, it becomes possible to predict prices, quantities, and other variables determined by the interaction of supply and demand at each level of the system.

In other words, given a set of estimates of the factors that affect the demand for and supply of dental care, an econometric model enables one to simulate the outcomes of the market such that estimates are derived for prices, utilization, and so forth. With a different set of assumptions regarding the demand and supply factors, new solutions for prices and quantities would be generated by the model. Thus the model enables us to follow throughout the system the effects of a change — for example, in the supply of dentists.

An econometric model is a system of mathematical equations that describe the interrelationships among the various markets of the dental (or any other) sector. Actual construction of a model involves a combination of subjective and objective decisions on the part of the model builder. Because it is necessary to describe the dental sector by a set of equations, it is necessary to be somewhat abstract and provide only a skeletal description of the many interrelationships that exist. However, the ability of these set of equations, once they have been statistically estimated, to be able to predict the desired variables in a consistent manner gives us some confidence both in the structure of the model and in the estimated relationships.

An econometric model applied to the dental sector has three basic uses, each of which is related to the interrelatedness of the system of equations. First, the model enables us to estimate dental utilization and prices (hence total expenditures on dental care) as a result of changes in income, population, or (given a more complete model than we have) a change in any demand factor. Similarly, it should be possible to conduct such simulations under varying supply conditions.

The second use of the model is for evaluating alternative policies. The model enables the user to make comparisons of the results of alternative policies proposed on either the demand or the supply side. For example, if it were desired to increase the amount of care received by the public, alternative policies might be suggested to reach this goal. On the supply side, the supply of dental care could be increased either by increasing the dentist input (e.g., increasing the number of dental school graduates via subsidizing the construction of new school capacity and providing loans and scholarships to students) or by increasing the productivity of the dentist-auxiliary "mix" (e.g., lessening the restrictions on the functions auxiliaries can perform, thus enabling them to perform tasks formerly done only by the dentist); on the demand side, the ability of consumers to obtain care could be increased by instituting a national dental health insurance program. Using the econometric model for this type of analysis, a comparison of the effects of each of these policies on price, quantity, and total expenditures, in relation to their costs, can be made. On the basis of these comparisons, the trade-offs between different policies become more apparent. Several such policy simulations will be undertaken in order to illustrate the usefulness of the model.

The third use of the model is to suggest those areas in which socioeconomic research should be undertaken in order to have the highest payoffs. Sensitivity analysis, which involves substituting different values for the parameters of the model and then observing the change in the variables being forecasted, enables us to determine which parts of the model are more important for determining the final outcomes, prices, utilization, etc. Research directed to these more sensitive areas will lead to refinements in those areas of the model which increase the accuracy of the expected results. A sensitivity analysis of the dental model has been included as Appendix 5B.

A Description of the Model

The dental sector has been theoretically specified at three levels: the market for dental visits; the market for dental manpower; and the market for dental manpower training facilities. In the first of these markets, the demand for visits is expected to be primarily related to price, income, population, age, sex, education, and fluoridation. The demand for care is expected to vary directly with income, population, and education; to vary inversely with the price of care and existence of fluoridation; and to be curvilinear (inverse "u") in its relationship to age.

The supply side of this market is expected to be a function of the price of a visit, the number of dentists (which acts as an overall constraint on the supply of dental care), and on the wages or prices that the dentist (in his role as entrepreneur) must pay for his inputs, such as for auxiliaries and equipment. The number of visits supplied is expected to vary directly with the number of dentists and the price of dental care, and vary inversely with the price of the inputs. Underlying this supply side is a production function, an equation which describes the amount of dental care that can be provided by different combinations of the dental inputs − that is, dental hours, the number and type of auxiliaries employed, and the type of equipment used.

Unfortunately, due to lack of data it was not possible to include all these variables in our model. As a result, only per capita income and the price per visit were included as determinants of demand, and only the number of dentists and price per visit were included as determinants of supply. It was also difficult, again because of data problems, to have a complete manpower sector to our model; consequently our dental care model consists only of levels one (visits) and three (training facilities). Even in these areas, further limitations have been imposed by lack of data. Originally we hoped to conduct separate cross sectional analyses for each of the survey periods, and, as subsequent survey data were gathered, to test and update the econometric model. Much of the necessary data has been gathered by the American Dental Association, but was unfortunately not made available to us in a less aggregated form than that published. It would be useful, in the interest of future research in this area, if this data would be either made available by the ADA or collected by some other organization which would then release it.[1]

The following are the estimated demand and supply equations for the dental services sector:

$$D_{VTh} = 1302.40 - 258.97 P_V + 1.22 Y \qquad (1a)$$
$$\text{(t-statistic)} \qquad\qquad (9.46) \qquad (14.25)$$
$$R^2 = .85$$

$$S_{VTh} = -804.20 + 66.32 P_V + 3535.10 DTh \qquad (2a)$$
$$\text{(t-statistic)} \qquad\qquad (4.58) \qquad (17.52)$$
$$R^2 = .90$$

D_{Vth} and S_{Vth} are the demand and supply of dental visits per thousand population, P_V is the price of a dental visit, Y is per capita income, and DTh is the number of dentists per thousand population. The results, which were estimated using two-stage least squares, are highly significant and have the expected signs. Demand for dental care varies directly with income and inversely with the price of dental care; the supply of dental care varies directly with both the stock of dentists and the price of care.

When the supply and demand equations are in log form, in order to more readily observe the elasticities of each variable, the equations are:

$$\text{Log } D_{VTh} = -1.15139 - 1.43 \text{ Log } P_V + 1.71 \text{ Log } Y \qquad (1b)$$

$$\text{(t-statistic)} \qquad\qquad (9.79) \qquad\quad (14.72)$$

$$R^2 = .86$$

$$\text{Log } S_{VTh} = 3.24701 + .29 \text{ Log } P_V + 1.08 \text{ Log } DTh \qquad (2b)$$

$$\text{(t-statistic)} \qquad\qquad (3.80) \qquad\quad (19.37)$$

$$R^2 = .92$$

Thus we observe that the demand for visits is both price and income elastic, while the supply of visits is inelastic with respect to price and elastic with respect to the long-run supply of dentists.

The second level of the dental care sector, the demand for and supply of dental manpower, is theoretically derived from the demand for and supply of dental services. The demand for manpower is thus determined by the demand for dental visits and the price (wage) of each type of manpower, relative to the price of other inputs. The supply of manpower is expected to be determined by its price (the incomes of both dentists and auxiliaries), relative to the wage in other professions into which a prospective dentist or auxiliary might enter; and by the cost to the prospective dentist/auxiliary of his training. In reality, the supply of manpower is primarily constrained by the supply of training facilities. A higher wage offered to dentists cannot, within conceivable limits, call forth more dentists than there are dental school spaces in which to produce them. Therefore the supply of dentists has been estimated as a function of the total number of dentists, with additions due to new dental school graduates and losses due to death and retirement. These relations are shown in the following set of equations:

$$DTh = DTh_{-1} + \Delta DTh \qquad (3)$$

$$\Delta DTh = GTh - RTh \qquad (4)$$

$$RTh = .02 \, DTh_{-1} \qquad (5)$$

$$GTh = ETh_{-1} - PTh_{\Sigma 4} \qquad (6)$$

$$PTh_{\Sigma 4} = .10 \, ETh_{-4} \qquad (7)$$

where DTh is the number of dentists per thousand population and (according to equation 3) this is equal to the number of dentists in the previous year (DTh_{-1})

and the change in the number of dentists (ΔDTh). The change in dentists (equation 4) is equal to the number of new dental graduates (GTh), less those dentists who die or retire (RTh), which in turn is related to the existing stock of dentists (DTh_{-1}). The number of dental graduates per thousand population (GTh) is equal to the number of entrants four years ago (ETh_{-4}), less those who have dropped out ($PTh_{\Sigma 4}$), which is in turn related to the number of dental school entrants (ETh_{-4}).

The demand for and supply of dental manpower training facilities — the third level of the model — is theoretically derived from the second level, the demand for and supply of dental manpower. In reality, the market for dental education is almost entirely determined on its supply side. In a freely operating market the amount of education available would vary directly with its price (tuition charges), but in actuality the determination of tuition is not jointly determined and is also not a determinant of the supply of educational capacity. We have reflected this in the specification of the market for dental school training, where the number of dental school entrants (ETh) is equal to dental school spaces (STh). The number of dental school spaces reflects the reality that the capacity of dental schools is the dominant constraint on the supply of dentist manpower.

$$ETh = STh \qquad (8)$$

$$STh = STh_{-1} + NSTh \qquad (9)$$

$$NSTh = \frac{Sub + MATCH}{\$308,000} \div \frac{Pop}{1000} \qquad (10)$$

Therefore the number of dental school spaces are equal to existing spaces (STh_{-1}) and additions to capacity (NSTh) as shown in equation 9. Additions to capacity (NSTh) are, as shown in equation 10, linearly related to the amount of construction subsidy funds (and matching, if required) available. $308,000 represents the average construction cost per dental place based on data from the Health Professions Education Act.

These sets of equations, then, are our model of the dental sector. The equations have been set up to allow one to trace the effects of subsidy funds on the supply of dentists and thus ultimately on the supply and price of dental care. Tracing these equations through from dental school capacity to the price and quantity of dental care, one sees that dental school spaces are the dominant constraint on the supply of dental manpower, since there are always more applicants than spaces. After net additions and subtractions to the number of dentists are taken into account, the new total number of dentists is then inserted into the demand and supply of visits equations, and thus their influence on price and quantity of dental care can be determined.

For ease in calculating the effects on price and quantity of dental visits, the reduced form equations,[a] which are derived by solving simultaneously the dental care demand and supply equations for price and quantity, will be used. These are:

$$P_V = 6.48 + .004Y - 10.87DTH \qquad (11)$$

$$V_{TH} = -374.70 + .25Y + 2814.37DTH \qquad (12)$$

The reduced form equations show that the price of dental care varies directly with income and inversely with the number of dentists; the supply of care varies directly with both income and the number of dentists.

Because "stock" variables (visits, dentists, dental school spaces, etc.) are on a per thousand population basis in the model (Th), the effects of population changes can be determined by multiplying these variables by the population in thousands. Total expenditures for dental care can be determined by multiplying the price per visit times total visits (which is determined by visits per thousand population times population in thousands).

One shortcoming of this econometric model lies in the fact that there is no precise, mathematical means by which to measure the effects on price and quantity of a change in the productivity of dentists, productivity of some other input, or relative factor mix of inputs. Ideally, we would like to have a production function which would show the effects on dentists' productivity (measured in terms of mean annual patient visits per dentist) of each of the inputs into the provision of dental care, such as dentist's time, auxiliary time, and capital equipment, such as chairs or high speed drills.

If there are changes in the amount of any input used, then the value of that variable would be increased by an appropriate amount; changes in the productivity of any input would be handled by an appropriate adjustment in its coefficient. For example, if a technological discovery resulted in the development of equipment that was 10 percent more efficient than existing equipment, and 50 percent of all dentists acquired the new equipment, the coefficient of the relevant capital variable could be increased by 5 percent to show the effects of the change on the mean annual patient visits that dentists are capable of providing.

The effects of any of these changes would be manifested in a change in the dependent variable of the production function — visits per dentist. One could then calculate the percentage change in this variable, and change the coefficient of dentists per thousand in the supply of care equation by an equal percentage

---

[a]The model consists of three endogenous variable (D_{VTh}, S_{VTh}, and P_V) in two equations (demand and supply for dental care). This is a system which cannot, mathematically, have a unique solution. However, when the market is in equilibrium, visits supplied will equal visits demanded at a particular price. Thus, for an equilibrium solution $D_{VTh} = S_{VTh}$ and there is now an equal number of equations and endogenous variables. The solution of this set of equations for P_V and V_{Th} are called the "reduced forms."

to reflect the change in overall dentist productivity (in the ability of the dentist and his "team" to provide services). Finally, the demand and supply equations would be re-solved for price of care and quantity of care (i.e., the reduced forms would be recalculated), so that the effect of the change in dentist productivity on those variables could be determined.

Due to data limitations we have been unable to estimate a production function for this model. Therefore, without a production function, our only means of allowing for the effects of change in use or productivity of an input is to make an educated guess as to how the change will affect overall dentist productivity, then make an appropriate adjustment in the coefficient of DTh in the supply of care equation, and finally, recalculate the reduced form equations.

Although we have not been able to estimate a production function, an estimate of one such function, by Alex Maurizi, is available, and in the analysis to follow we will make use of both methods for allowing for changes in productivity.[2] This production function, as estimated by Maurizi (in logarithms) is:

$$Ln\,(VPD) = 1.446 + .466\,Ln\,(AUX) + .777\,Ln\,(HRD) + .254\,Ln\,(CHR)$$
$$R^2 = .31 \tag{13}$$

where VPD = annual patient visits per dentist; AUX = number of full-time auxiliaries employed by a dentist; HRD = number of annual hours worked by a dentist; CHR = number of chairs in the office.

Having described the specification, construction, and estimation of the dental care sector model (as well as its limitations) we will now illustrate the use of the model for forecasting and policy analysis.

Forecasting with an Econometric Model

Traditional techniques used in the dental field for estimating future dental requirements center around the use of personnel-to-population (usually the dentist-to-population) ratios. The current year ratio is generally used to measure the current provision of services by dentists, and the maintenance of this ratio in a future year, given a certain population projection, is usually the desired goal. Implicit in the use of the ratio technique is the assumption that maintaining the existing dentist-population ratio is desirable and that it maintains an "equilibrium" situation. An estimate is then made of the likely supply of dentists in the target year, with subtractions made from the existing stock for deaths and retirements, and additions as a result of graduates from existing and new dental schools. Finally, there is a comparison between dentist manpower "needs" and "supply" in the target year, with the difference usually being negative, i.e., additions to the supply of dentists are required if the base year ratio is to be maintained.

The econometric model differs in several important respects from the ratio technique. First, there are normative implications in the model itself — it merely attempts to predict the values of certain variables under varying conditions. Thus forecasts using the econometric model are "neutral" in their goal implications. Second, the model as developed by economists realizes that the demand by the public is not for dentists, but for dental care measured in terms of visits. The demand for dentists is thus derived from the initial demand for dental visits. In this framework the dentist is viewed as being not the only input into the production of a dental visit; equipment and auxiliary personnel are also important. Thus the "need" for dentists may depend not only on the public's demand for dental visits but also upon the other inputs and the extent to which it is possible to use them.

Based upon the model, therefore, the forecast of the supply of dental care is also viewed in terms of visits rather than dentists, and the supply of visits is determined not only upon the expected supply of dentists but also upon the price per visit, with adjustments in the coefficient of dentists per thousand for expected changes in dentist productivity. In a more complete model, the expected values of other variables such as the price of inputs would also be considered in forecasting the available supply of visits in the target year.

Third, the economic approach attempts to estimate the demand rather than the need for dental care and it recognizes that the demand for care is not constant throughout the population. Demand for visits is forecast based upon estimates of personal income and price per visit (and population, if the equations are converted from a per thousand to an absolute basis) in the target year. In a more complete model, of course, estimates of other variables such as fluoridation, age distribution, and education would also be incorporated into the forecast.

It would therefore be highly unlikely that maintenance of a dentist-population ratio would be an accurate indication of the number of dentists "needed" for some future period. Although a given dentist-population ratio may represent the situation that currently exists, the demand for dental care is likely to increase in the future; therefore, the maintenance of the same ratio is likely to result in too few dentists at current prices thus resulting in higher prices for dental care (other things being unchanged). Further, the productivity of dentists is likely to continue to change; the supply of visits from a given number of dentists will therefore be greater in the future than at present. Maintenance of a given dentist-population ratio in this latter instance will result in either more dentists than demanded, at the same price of a visit, or it may result in less of an increase in dentist productivity, so as to enable dentists to work as many hours as they would like.

For a given population, therefore, it is highly unlikely that the demand and supply of dental care in some future period will be the same as it is at present. A new equilibrium situation will occur by adjustments being made in the price of dental care. If the increase in demand for care resulting from increases in population or per capita income has been greater than the increase in supply resulting from productivity changes or numbers of dentists, then the price of dental care will rise. Implicit in the dentist-population technique is that a constant dentist-population ratio results in the *same* price of dental care that currently exists. Increases in the supply of dentists presumably assume no demand or productivity changes, thus maintaining the price of dental care.

It is in this way that forecasting leads us toward formulating and comparing alternative policies. By forecasting both demand and supply with the econometric model we will be able to predict the future price of dental care. Given this estimate of the price of dental care we can then determine alternative ways of reducing it (if so desired), either by increasing supply (again in alternative ways) or by reducing the price of care for certain population groups (a demand subsidy). A difficulty with the methodology underlying the ratio technique is that it suggests limited policy alternatives, i.e., changes in the supply of dentists. Also, the ratio technique does not allow the objective to be clearly stated; for example, does the maintenance of a dentist-population ratio have a redistribution objective? Thus, forecasting outcomes in the dental sector with an econometric model is not directly comparable with results based on use of the ratio technique, which, by estimating requirements for dentists, is more of a value judgment with respect to goals for dentists.

As an example of the use of the econometric model, we will forecast the market for dental care in 1975 and compare these outcomes to those which would occur when a constant dentist-population ratio is maintained. Since the ratio technique and the econometric model are not directly comparable for forecasting purposes, why compare forecasts of the dental sector based on these two approaches? First, to illustrate the additional information that the model provides regarding future outcomes and second, to show, in terms of these outcomes, what the implications are of maintaining a constant dentist-population ratio.

The variables to be forecast are: the price of a visit, visits per thousand population (and total visits), total expenditures on dental care, and dentists' incomes — assuming they receive a certain percentage of future dental expenditures. In order to make these forecasts we will need some estimates of the number of dentists, the population, and personal incomes in 1975. For simplicity, we will use as our estimate for number of dentists in 1975 the projection made by the Department of Health, Education, and Welfare — 111,400. Both a "high" and a "low" estimate will be used for per capita income ($4,281 and $4,510) and for population (213,800,000 and 218,000,000) in 1975. We could have used our own estimate of dental supply using the dental school-dental manpower sector of the model. However, since we wished to make some forecasts with a given supply of dentists, it is not important whose estimate of dentists is used. In the next section we will forecast the supply of dentists under different policy alternatives and then incorporate these different numbers into our forecasts.

The reduced form equations for demand and supply of dental visits are:

$$P_V = 6.48 + .004Y - 10.87 DTh \qquad (11a)$$

$$V_{Th} = -374.70 + .25Y + 2814.37 DTh \qquad (12a)$$

Using the estimates of per capita income = $4,281, population = 213,800,000 and dentists = 111,400, we derive the following estimates for price and number of visits per thousand population:

$$P_V = 6.48 + .004(4281) - 10.87 \frac{111,400}{213,800} = \$17.94$$

$$V_{Th} = -374.70 + .25(4281) + 2814.37 \frac{111,400}{213,800} = 2159.02$$

Total visits are equal to 2159.02 (213,800) = 461,598,476 and total expenditures on dental care are equal to the price of a visit multiplied by the number of visits, which is $8,281,076,000.[3] If we assume that dentists' net income is equal to 53 percent of gross income (which is equal to total dental expenditures divided by the number of dentists), we arrive at an estimate of average annual dentist net income in 1975 of $39,398 [($8,281,076,000 X .53) ÷ 111,400].[4]

The results of these forecasts, for different assumptions of income and population, are summarized in Table 5-1. Another way of forecasting the above variables for 1975 is to indicate the percent increases that are expected in each of the forecast variables. This can easily be determined by using the reduced form equations in log form and inserting the percentage increases in income, population, and dentists and thus determining the percentage increases in prices and visits per thousand population. These reduced form equations, in logs, are:

$$\text{Log } P_V = 2.55621 + .99 \text{ Log } Y - .63 \text{ Log } DTh \qquad (11b)$$

$$\text{Log } D_{VTh} = 2.50541 + .29 \text{ Log } Y + .90 \text{ Log } DTh \qquad (12b)$$

The percentage increases from 1970 to 1975 in the above variables are presented in Table 5-2.

These forecasts indicate that even without any national insurance plan for dental care we can expect higher prices and hence increased expenditures for dental care in 1975. Visits will also increase, but their percentage increase will be smaller, than the percentage increases in prices and expenditures. The difference in total expenditures between the low and the high estimate of both income and population is almost one billion dollars. Dentists' average net incomes, under these ranges of estimates, are expected to be from 38.5 to 51.3 percent higher in 1975 than in 1970.

Table 5-1. Forecasts of Prices, Visits, Expenditures, and Dental Incomes in 1975

	P_V	VTh	Total Visits	Total Expenditures	Dentists Income
Per Capita Income (4281) Population (213,800)	$17.94	2159.02	461,498,476	$8,281,076,000	$39,398
Per Capita Income (4510) Population (213,800)	18.86	2216.27	473,838,526	8,936,594,000	42,517
Per Capita Income (4281) Population (218,000)	18.05	2130.88	464,531,840	8,384,799,000	39,892
Per Capita Income (4510) Population (218,000)	18.97	2188.13	477,012,340	9,048,924,090	43,051

The forecasts also illustrate the general expectations under which the model was specified. The demand for visits varies directly with income and inversely with price; the supply of visits varies directly with both price and number of dentists. As population is increased with a constant dentist supply, visits per thousand population decrease and price increases, although total visits and total expenditures both increase. Increasing income with a constant population results in an increase in visits per thousand, total visits, price, and total expenditures for dental care.

In order to compare the forecasting results of the econometric model when a constant population-dentist ratio is maintained, let us assume that the result of using a ratio technique would be the maintenance in 1975 of the 1970 population-dentist ratio.[5] In 1970 the population-dentist ratio was 1:1,966 (or .51 dentists per thousand population). If the goal was merely to maintain this ratio into 1975, what would be the consequences? If we refer back to Tables 5-1 and 5-2, the high population estimate for 1975 (218,000,000) would give us approximately the same population-dentist ratio as in 1970 (it would actually be slightly more favorable, 1:1,956). Thus even maintaining the same population-dentist ratio, the price of dental care would still be 25 to 31 percent greater than in 1970 because of increased demands for dental care, as indicated by the higher estimate of per capita income.

Since dental care is income elastic — that is, increases in per capita incomes are likely to cause greater than proportionate increases in dental care utilization — any policy aimed at merely maintaining a dentist-population ratio that existed in the past will not indicate what the price of dental care will be in the future. If prices for care are higher, the amount of dental care demanded will be lower, particularly for the lower income groups. One must therefore question the implicit objectives of using dentist-population ratios for estimating future dental supply requirements.

Table 5-2. Forecasts of the Percent Increase in Prices, Visits, Expenditures, and Dental Incomes, 1970-1975

Percent Increase	Percent Increase in P_V	Percent Increase in VTH	Percent Increase in Total Visits	Percent Increase in Total Expenditures	Percent Increase in Dentists' Income
Income (27.4) Population (4.9)	24.7	13.6	19.2	48.9	38.5
Income (34.2) Population (4.9)	31.1	16.6	22.4	60.7	49.4
Income (27.4) Population (7.0)	25.4	12.1	20.0	50.8	40.2
Income (34.2) Population (7.0)	31.8	15.1	23.2	62.7	51.3

The above forecasts for 1975 demonstrate the differences between the ratio technique and the econometric model for forecasting purposes. The dentist-population ratio technique makes no allowance for increases in demand resulting from causes other than population growth, such as increases in incomes, prepaid dental care plans, or changes in the age distribution. The econometric model, however, attempts to incorporate such demand factors when forecasting future demand for dental care. Second, the ratio technique approaches the demand for care in terms of the demand for dentists; the econometric approach attempts to forecast the demand for visits. (A more refined analysis, data permitting, would be to separate out dental visits into its various components, e.g., fillings, extractions, etc.) As will be discussed in the next section on policy analysis, this difference in estimating demand for dental care in terms of dentists versus visits suggests alternative approaches toward increasing utilization of dental care. The supply of dentists is viewed as only one of several inputs into the production of dental visits. Thus the forecasted demand for care does not necessarily have to be met by a specific supply of dentists, as is assumed by the ratio technique. Instead the model tells us the forecasted demand for care can be provided through a variety of technologically and legally feasible combinations of dentists, auxiliaries, and capital equipment. Thus, a different approach is also used for forecasting the likely supply of care.

Finally, the econometric model enables the forecaster to present (in addition to demand and supply estimates) estimates of future prices, expenditures, and visits under different assumptions. The ratio technique estimates a gap between the need for and the likely supply of dentists, but does not provide any information as to what this gap means in terms of higher prices, or fewer visits. How then is one able to place a value on eliminating a gap of 1,000 or 10,000 dentists?

Once forecasts have been made, policy alternatives are then usually formulated in order to bring about changes in the predicted outcomes. The next section will continue the application of the econometric model for purposes of evaluating policy alternatives.

Policy Analysis Using an Econometric Model

A demonstration of the use of the econometric model for purposes of policy analysis follows naturally from the demonstration of its use in forecasting. Forecasts of anticipated needs for and supply of dental services are usually followed by policy recommendations designed to narrow the forecasted gap between these anticipated needs and projected supplies. Because forecasts, traditionally made using a ratio technique, generally center on the desired quantity and the actual supply of dentists, the follow-up policy proposals based on this approach usually center on increasing the supply of dentists through increasing dental school capacity. Forecasts using an econometric model, however, indicate that changes in the forecasted values of utilization and prices can be affected through many factors that effect both demand and supply. If the goal was to increase utilization of dental services then this could be achieved by either increasing the demand for dental care by subsidizing the purchase of dental care, or by lowering the price of dental care through subsidies on the supply side, hence increasing utilization. Note, however, that the true price of a unit of dental care would rise in either case. If, for example, the desired policy was instead to lower or maintain the prevailing price of dental care, then demand could be decreased by instituting fluoridation, hence with less demand the price of care will be lower than it would be otherwise. The econometric model is thus a tool for the policy maker to use for evaluating and comparing alternatives. Predictions can be made of the outcomes of policies in terms of increased visits, price changes, and comparisons of the money cost and benefits of these alternatives can be made.

Redistribution and efficiency are the two major roles for government in the dental area; these are discussed more fully in Chapter 6. To use the model for comparing policy alternatives let us assume that with regard to the personal dental services sector, the goal (which is a value judgment) is redistributive; further, that it is meant to be redistribution in kind (i.e., to increase the use of dental care by some population group); and that the government would like to achieve this redistribution at minimum cost. Increased utilization can be achieved by subsidizing the demand or the supply of dental care. One comparison that should therefore be made is the relative cost of increasing utilization through subsidies on either the demand or the supply side. Further, since there are alternative means of increasing the supply of dental services, a comparison of their relative costs will be undertaken.

There are three methods by which supply can be increased: (1) an increase in the number of dentists; (2) an increase in dental productivity, using auxiliaries with the same set of tasks currently allowed; and (3) lowering restrictions on tasks performed by auxiliaries so that dental productivity can be increased even more. The first two of these supply policies will be analyzed and compared.

Increases in the Number of Dentists

Policies to increase the number of dentists are similar to the intent underlying the Health Professions Education Act (HPEA), therefore an analysis of the cost as well as the consequences of a larger number of dentists should involve an attempt to analyze the past as well as the probable future performance of the HPEA. To accomplish this a simulation of the HPEA using the econometric model was undertaken.

Since the HPEA did not actually begin until 1965, we did not begin the simulation until that year. For the years 1965-1971 we used the actual HPEA construction expenditures for each year as the value for subsidy (SUB). Matching funds (MATCH) were assumed to be one-half of subsidy (SUB) since the program was set up on a 2/3-1/3 federal funds-matching funds basis. For simplicity we assumed that each year's expenditures resulted in new dental school spaces in the same year in which they were spent. In reality, of course, there was certainly a lag, not to mention the fact that each year's expenditure totals represent the monies which the government made a commitment to spend in that year but say nothing about when the money was actually spent. Thus in our simulation the effects of any particular expenditures are probably felt before they actually resulted in new places. Finally, the coefficient in the model for construction funds on new dental school spaces (1/$308,000) is based on the actual cost per space of spaces constructed under HPEA aid over 1965-1971. Additional expenditures for student and institutional support have also been shown in order to calculate the total yearly cost of the program.

For the first few years of the HPEA program we used actual lagged values when necessary; once the model began to generate new values these were used in the simulation. For example, for the years 1965-1968 "dental graduates" were based on the actual values of "dental entrants" for 1961-1964, before program expenditures actually began. In 1969 we were able to base the "dental graduates" on our calculated value of "dental entrants" in 1965.

When the HPEA program was projected to 1975, the estimates for subsidy (SUB) were based on the average of the actual expenditures for 1970-1971. Two population and income forecasts were used for 1975; one was based on the low estimates of income and population and the other on the high estimates of income and population used in the previous section on forecasting.

When the HPEA program was proposed in 1962 the estimates for population, number of dentists, and cost per dentist were quite different from what actually occurred. The accuracy of the original estimates have been discussed earlier; in this section we wish to examine the effects of the program, therefore actual data are used in the analysis. Table 5-3 shows the data used in the yearly simulations of the HPEA. The total federal yearly cost of the HPEA program is at the bottom of the table, while at the top are the outcomes of the simulations in terms of price per visit, visits per thousand population, total visits, total expenditures, and average net incomes of dentists.

In order to indicate the effect that the HPEA has had on these outcome measures, another simulation was conducted which assumed that there was no HPEA program, resulting in fewer dental spaces. The number of new dental spaces each year without the HPEA was estimated to be the average number of new entrants to dental schools in the preceeding five-year period, which was approximately 55 per year. The outcomes of this simulation are shown in Table 5-4. Additional simulations were conducted for the period 1971-1975. One set of simulations was based on the assumptions that the HPEA program would continue at its 1970-1971 funding. A simulation under this assumption was then run using the low estimates of income and population for 1971-1975; and then

Table 5-3. A Simulation of the Health Professions Education Act, 1964-1971

		1964	1965	1966	1967	1968	1969	1970	1971
	DDSY	$ 17,675	$ 19,278	$ 20,873	$ 22,531	$ 24,602	$ 26,445	$ 28,974	$ 31,629
(000's)	TE	3,088,079	3,399,516	3,736,867	4,096,403	4,543,015	4,961,003	5,522,519	6,131,055
(000's)	TV	296,077	310,091	322,520	335,357	350,099	363,901	380,765	398,439
	VTH	1549.45	1602.87	1649.71	1699.09	1756.54	1807.70	1868.92	1935.75
	PV	10.43	10.96	11.57	12.22	12.98	13.63	14.50	15.39
	Y	2,293	2,441	2,603	2,768	2,966	3,138	3,361	3,591
	DTH	.4846	.4858	.4881	.4910	.4938	.4967	.4986	.5020
	POP	191,085	193,460	195,501	197,374	199,312	201,306	203,736	205,832
	DDS	92,597	93,990	95,422	96,906	98,421	99,989	101,592	103,319
	ΔD	+845	+1,393	+1,432	+1,484	+1,514	+1,568	+1,603	+1,728
	R	2,368	1,852	1,880	1,908	1,938	1,968	2,000	2,032
	DDS_{-1}	91,752	92,597	93,990	95,422	96,906	98,421	99,989	101,592
	G	3,213	3,245	3,312	3,393	3,452	3,537	3,602	3,760
	$P_{\Sigma 4}$	403	360	368	377	384	393	400	418
	E_{-4}	3,836	3,605	3,680	3,770	3,836	3,930	4,003	4,117
	E	3,836	3,930	4,003	4,177	4,292	4,410	4,554	4,686
	S	3,836	3,930	4,003	4,177	4,292	4,410	4,554	4,686
	S_{-1}	3,770	3,836	3,930	4,003	4,177	4,292	4,410	4,554
	NS	66	94	73	174	115	118	144	132
(000's)	MATCH	0	9,620	7,499	17,931	11,785	12,083	14,821	13,549
(000's)	SUB	0	19,240	14,997	35,862	23,570	24,186	29,642	27,098
(000's)	Other Dollars[1]	0	2,871	7,599	16,381	19,850	27,068	28,645	33,040
(000's)	Total Dollars	0	31,731	30,095	70,173	55,205	63,337	73,108	74,087
(000's)	Total Federal Subsidy Dollars	0	22,111	22,597	52,242	43,420	51,254	58,287	60,538

1. Student plus Institutional Support.

Table 5-4. A Simulation Without HPEA, 1964-1971

		1964	1965	1966	1967	1968	1969	1970	1971
DDSY	(000's)	$ 17,675	$ 19,278	$ 20,873	$ 22,531	$ 24,603	$ 26,451	$ 28,989	$ 31,675
TE	(000's)	3,088,079	3,399,516	3,736,867	4,096,403	4,543,015	4,960,350	5,520,770	6,125,651
TV		296,077	310,091	322,520	335,357	350,099	363,803	380,525	397,757
VTH		1549.45	1602.87	1649.71	1699.09	1756.54	1807.21	1867.74	1932.44
PV		10.43	10.96	11.57	12.22	12.98	13.63	14.51	15.50
Y		2,293	2,441	2,603	2,768	2,966	3,138	3,361	3,591
DTH		.4846	.4858	.4881	.4910	.4938	.4965	.4982	.5008
POP		191,085	193,460	195,501	197,374	199,312	210,306	203,736	205,832
DDS		92,597	93,990	95,422	96,906	98,421	99,954	101,506	103,077
ΔD		+845	+1,393	+1,432	+1,485	+1,514	+1,533	+1,552	+1,571
R		2,368	1,852	1,880	1,908	1,938	1,968	1,999	2,030
DDS_{-1}		91,752	92,597	93,990	95,422	96,906	98,421	99,954	101,506
G		3,213	3,245	3,312	3,343	3,452	3,502	3,551	3,601
$P_{\Sigma 4}$		403	360	368	377	384	389	395	400
$E_{\Sigma 4}$		3,616	3,605	3,680	3,770	3,836	3,891	3,946	4,001
E_{-4}		3,836	3,891	3,946	4,001	4,056	4,111	4,166	4,221
S		3,836	3,891	3,946	4,001	4,056	4,111	4,166	4,221
$\bar{S}_{-1}$		3,770	3,836	3,891	3,946	4,001	4,056	4,111	4,166
NS		66	55	55	55	55	55	55	55

one using the high income and population estimates. These are shown in Tables 5-5 and 5-6. Another set of simulations continued the earlier assumption of no HPEA program and a simulation was run under each of the income and population estimates; these are shown in Tables 5-7 and 5-8.

As seen from Table 5-3, although federal expenditures under the HPEA started in 1965, an increase in the number of graduates did not come about for several years. Because of continuing increases in demand, the projected price of dental care continued to rise as did the number of visits per thousand population. The projected dentist-population ratio continued to increase throughout this period: from .48 per 1,000 population in 1964, to .50 per 1,000 population in 1971, and .52 per 1,000 population in 1975. For comparative purposes, the following series are equivalent:

Dentist/Population Ratio	Population: Dentist Ratio
.46 (per 1,000 population)	2174:1
.48	2084:1
.50	2000:1
.52	1923:1
.54	1852:1
.56	1786:1
.58	1725:1

Over the period of the HPEA, from 1965 to 1971, the simulations with and without the HPEA show that differences in all the outcome variables are very slight and occur only in the latter years. The price per visit is less than 1 percent lower in 1969 and 1970 and the number of visits are also only slightly higher, approximately 0.1 percent as result of the HPEA program. Total expenditures on dental care are approximately two million dollars a year lower in 1969 and 1970 without the HPEA.

When the HPEA program was endorsed by the dental profession it was requested for a ten-year period, to end in 1975. However it is now scheduled to continue until at least 1980. Since the accuracy of both population and income forecasts is so questionable that far into the future, comparisons have only been made until 1975. (One could, however, continue the simulations into 1980 under various estimates of population and income.)

The differences between the simulations with and without the HPEA become slightly more noticeable the further one goes into the future. The dentist-population ratio is .51 per 1,000 population with HPEA versus .50 per 1,000 population without the HPEA using the estimates of high income and high population (HY, HP), while it is .52 per 1,000 population to .51 per 1,000 population, respectively, under the lower population and income estimates (LY, LP). Both of these are greater than the dentist population ratio that prevailed before the HPEA. Differences in price per visit are still small: $19.06 versus $18.99, respectively (HY, HP). Utilization and utilization rates are approximately 1 percent higher by 1975 under the HPEA program. Since utilization has

Table 5-5. HPEA Simulation, 1972-1975: Low Income and Low Population Forecasts

		1972	1973	1974	1975
	DDSY	$ 33,616	$ 35,648	$ 37,692	$ 39,771
(000's)	TE	6,629,644	7,155,181	7,704,025	8,281,125
(000's)	TV	413,474	428,929	444,771	461,049
	VTH	1989.54	2044.31	2099.78	2156.45
	PV	16.03	16.68	17.32	17.96
	Y	3,763	3,936	4,108	4,281
	DTH	.5058	.5099	.5143	.5191
	POP	207,824	209,816	211,818	213,800
	DDS	105,116	106,982	108,942	110,980
	ΔD	+1,797	+1,867	+1,959	+2,039
	R	2,066	2,102	2,140	2,179
	DDS_{-1}	103,319	105,116	106,982	108,942
	G	3,863	3,969	4,099	4,218
	$P_{\Sigma 4}$	429	441	455	469
	E_{-4}	4,292	4,410	4,554	4,686
	E	4,823	4,959	5,095	5,232
	S	4,823	4,959	5,095	5,232
	S_{-1}	4,686	4,823	4,959	5,095
	NS	137	136	136	137
(000's)	MATCH	14,000	14,000	14,000	14,000
(000's)	SUB	28,000	28,000	28,000	28,000
(000's)	Other Dollars[1]	30,000	30,000	30,000	30,000
(000's)	Total Dollars	72,000	72,000	72,000	72,000
(000's)	Total Federal Subsidy	58,000	58,000	58,000	58,000

1. Student plus Institutional Support.

increased by a greater percentage than the percentage decline in the price of a visit, annual expenditures on dental care are 40-43 million dollars a year greater with the HPEA program. If the simulations were conducted further into the future, one would expect such trends to continue.[6]

Alternative Policies for Increasing the Supply of Dental Care

Through 1971 the cost of the HPEA had been approximately 350 million dollars; further, it was expected to continue at a federal subsidy of 58 million dollars a year. Assuming that the objective of this program was to achieve an increase in supply of dental care, one might ask whether an equivalent increase in supply could have been achieved through alternative programs at a lower cost. One such alternative is shown. An additional table has been constructed (Table 5-9) that shows the increase in dental productivity that would be needed in order to provide the equivalent number of visits as provided under the HPEA program.

The first two lines in the table show the total visits in each year with and without the HPEA program, according to the simulations. These two visit totals

Table 5-6. HPEA Simulation, 1972-1975: High Income and High Population Forecasts

		1972	1973	1974	1975
	DDSY	$ 34,460	$ 37,380	$ 40,380	$ 43,445
(000's)	TE	6,796,025	7,502,819	8,253,425	9,045,994
(000's)	TV	417,097	436,301	456,116	476,450
	VTH	1996.88	2058.84	2121.88	2185.55
	PV	16.29	17.20	18.10	18.99
	Y	3,821	4,051	4,281	4,510
	DTH	.5033	.5048	.5068	.5091
	POP	208,874	211,916	214,958	218,000
	DDS	105,116	106,982	108,942	110,980
	ΔD	+1,797	+1,867	+1,959	+2,039
	R	2,066	2,102	2,140	2,179
	DDS_{-1}	103,319	105,116	106,982	108,942
	G	3,863	3,969	4,099	4,218
	$P_{\Sigma 4}$	429	441	455	469
	E_{-4}	4,292	4,410	4,554	4,686
	E	4,823	4,959	5,095	5,232
	S	4,823	4,959	5,095	5,232
	S_{-1}	4,686	4,823	4,959	5,095
	NS	137	136	136	137
(000's)	MATCH	14,000	14,000	14,000	14,000
(000's)	SUB	28,000	28,000	28,000	28,000
(000's)	Other Dollars[1]	30,000	30,000	30,000	30,000
(000's)	Total Dollars	72,000	72,000	72,000	72,000
(000's)	Total Federal Subsidy Dollars	58,000	58,000	58,000	58,000

1. Student plus Institutional Support.

are equal for years 1964-1968. This is due to the time lag involved in producing dentists; the original new spaces created by HPEA in 1965 do not produce their first new dentists until 1969. The total visit figures for some later years may be somewhat under- or overstated due to effects of rounding, so the figures for needed productivity increases may in those years be slightly over- or understated.

Line 3 shows the stock of active practicing dentists in each year, assuming no HPEA program. Mean annual patient visits per dentist for each year in the nonHPEA situation are shown in line 4. Line 5 shows how many patient visits per year each dentist in the nonHPEA case would have to provide if total visits in the nonHPEA case were to equal total visits in the HPEA case. Finally, line 6 gives the productivity increase dentists in the nonHPEA situation would have to make in each case in order to provide an amount of total visits equivalent to the amount for that year in the HPEA situation.

An estimate was made of the increase in the number of auxiliary personnel that would be required if the dentist's productivity were to be sufficient to provide the same number of visits as under the HPEA program. This estimate of

Table 5-7. Simulation, 1972-1975 Without HPEA: Low Income and Low Population Forecasts

		1972	1973	1974	1975
	DDSY	$ 33,707	$ 35,798	$ 37,923	$ 40,104
(000's)	TE	6,619,038	7,137,500	7,676,769	8,241,706
(000's)	TV	412,207	426,931	441,829	456,987
	VTH	1983.44	2034.79	2085.89	2137.45
	PV	16.06	16.72	17.37	18.03
	Y	3,763	3,936	4,108	4,281
	DTH	.5036	.5065	.5094	.5123
	POP	207,824	209,816	211,818	213,800
	DDS	104,666	106,272	107,896	109,537
	ΔD	+1,589	+1,607	+1,624	+1,641
	R	2,062	2,093	2,125	2,158
	DDS_{-1}	103,077	104,666	106,272	107,896
	G	3,650	3,700	3,749	3,799
	$P_{\Sigma 4}$	406	411	417	422
	E_{-4}	4,056	4,111	4,166	4,221
	E	4,276	4,331	4,386	4,441
	S	4,276	4,331	4,386	4,441
	S_{-1}	4,221	4,276	4,331	4,386
	NS	55	55	55	55

Table 5-8. Simulation, 1972-1975 Without HPEA: High Income and High Population Forecasts

		1972	1973	1974	1975
	DDSY	$ 34,553	$ 37,537	$ 40,627	$ 43,807
(000's)	TE	6,785,125	7,484,269	8,224,144	9,002,869
(000's)	TV	415,830	434,303	453,174	472,389
	VTH	1990.82	2049.41	2108.20	2166.92
	PV	16.32	17.23	18.15	19.06
	Y	3,821	4,051	4,281	4,510
	DTH	.5011	.5015	.5019	.5025
	POP	208,874	211,916	214,958	218,000
	DDS	104,666	106,272	107,896	109,537
	ΔD	+1,589	+1,607	+1,624	+1,641
	R	2,062	2,093	3,125	2,158
	DDS_{-1}	103,077	104,666	106,272	107,896
	G	3,650	3,700	3,749	3,799
	$P_{\Sigma 4}$	406	411	417	422
	E_{-4}	4,056	4,111	4,166	4,221
	E	4,276	4,331	4,386	4,441
	S	4,276	4,331	4,386	4,441
	S_{-1}	4,221	4,276	4,331	4,386
	NS	55	55	55	55

Table 5-9. Productivity Increases Needed in NonHPEA Situation to Provide Number of Visits Equivalent to HPEA Situation

		1964	1965	1966	1967	1968	1969	1970	1971
(000's)	Total Visits With HPEA	296,007	310,091	322,520	335,357	350,099	363,901	380,765	398,044
(000's)	Total Visits Without HPEA	296,007	310,091	322,520	335,357	350,099	363,803	380,525	397,757
	DDS Without HPEA	92,597	93,990	95,422	96,906	98,421	99,954	101,506	103,077
	VPD Without HPEA	3197.48	3299.19	3379.93	3460.64	3557.16	3639.70	3748.79	3858.83
	VPD Without HPEA necessary to Equal TV with HPEA	3197.48	3299.19	3379.93	3460.64	3557.16	3640.68	3751.16	3865.45
	Percent increase in productivity necessary without HPEA	00.00	00.00	00.00	00.00	00.00	00.03	00.06	00.17

additional auxiliary persons was made using the production function for dental services estimated by Alex Maurizi (see also Note 2).

Maurizi's production function is:

$$\text{Log VPD} = .62798 + .466 \text{ Log AUX} + .77 \text{ Log HRD} + .254 \text{ Log CHR}$$

Where VPD = mean annual patient visits per dentist; AUX = mean number of auxiliary personnel employed by dentists; HRD = mean annual hours worked per dentist; and CHR = mean number of chairs in the office. Thus, a 10 percent increase in the average number of auxiliaries per dentist would result in a 4.66 percent increase in visits per dentist (.466 X 10).

According to Table 5-9, it would have required an increase of 0.06 percent in dentist productivity in 1970 to equal the additional number of visits produced under the HPEA program. By 1975 (Table 5-10) it would have required an increase in productivity of approximately 0.9 percent. Therefore, the additional number of auxiliaries required in 1970 was:

$$\frac{0.06 \text{ (Percent increase in productivity)}}{.466 \text{ (coefficient of auxiliaries)}} = .13 \text{ percent}$$

while for 1975 it would have required:

$$\frac{0.9}{.466} = 1.93 \text{ percent}$$

In 1970 there were 145,200 auxiliaries in the United States (see Table 3-5). Since the supply of dentists in 1970 was 101,506, there were 1.4305 auxiliaries per dentist. In 1970 the increase in auxiliary utilization would have had to be .13 percent greater, therefore it would have required 1.4324 auxiliaries per dentist (1.4305 X 1.0013 = 1.4324 auxiliaries per dentist). The number of additional auxiliaries required would therefore had to have been 193 [(1.4324 − 1.4305) (101,506)]. The average wage of auxiliaries in 1970 was approximately $5,000.[7] Therefore the additional cost of these 193 auxiliaries would be approximately $965,000 per year. By 1975 the annual cost of the additional auxiliaries would be $21,000,000.[8]

The amounts represent the annual federal subsidies that would have to be paid to dentists in order to subsidize their use of auxiliaries. Conceptually, then, these annual subsidies for auxiliaries should be compared to the subsidies under the HPEA program. The timing of the expenditures and when they result in increased visits should also be considered. In this framework, if the objective of the HPEA program was viewed as desiring an increase in dental visits, it would have been less expensive (less than 10 percent of the cost) to subsidize the use of auxiliaries than to produce the equivalent number of visits through the HPEA program.

Table 5-10. Productivity Increases Needed in NonHPEA Situation to Provide Number of Visits Equivalent to HPEA Situation, 1972-1975

		1972	1973	1974	1975
Low Income and Low Population Forecasts					
(000's)	Total Visits with HPEA	413,474	428,929	444,771	461,049
(000's)	Total Visits without HPEA	412,207	426,931	441,829	456,987
	DDS without HPEA	104,666	106,272	107,896	109,537
	VPD without HPEA	3938.31	4017.34	4094.95	4171.99
	VPD without HPEA necessary to equal TV with HPEA	3950.41	4036.14	4122.22	4209.07
	Percent Increase in productivity necessary without HPEA	00.31	00.47	00.67	00.89
High Income and High Population Forecasts					
(000's)	Total Visits with HPEA	417,097	436,301	456,116	476,450
(000's)	Total Visits without HPEA	415,830	434,303	453,174	472,389
	DDS without HPEA	104,666	106,272	107,896	109,537
	VPD without HPEA	3972.92	4086.71	4200.10	4312.60
	VPD without HPEA necessary to equal TV with HPEA	3985.03	4105.51	4227.37	4349.67
	Percent Increase in productivity necessary without HPEA	00.30	00.46	00.65	00.86

From 1970-1975 the auxiliary subsidy program would cost between $53-55 million, depending upon whether the forecasts are based on low income-low population or high income-high population. The total federal dollars under the HPEA from 1965-1975 are estimated at $542 million. (Total dollars to include federal and matching funds are estimated at $686 million.) Based on a comparison of their present values, the auxiliary subsidy program would be even less than 10 percent of the HPEA cost.

There are of course a number of implicit assumptions underlying such a comparison and several of these should perhaps be noted. How effective would a subsidy program to dentists be for hiring auxiliaries? If the dentist is relatively unresponsive to working more hours as the price of a visit is increased (and the evidence cited earlier by us and Maurizi indicate it is very inelastic), and the dentists were interested in increased income — and further if the substitutability between dentists and auxiliaries in some of the tasks to be performed was good (there is much evidence in support of this, for example the article by Ruth Roemer, op. cit.) — then such a subsidy program for auxiliaries should be effective in achieving its objective. In fact it could be argued that such a subsidy might not even be needed, at least in full. If demand for dental care continues to increase, then the likely response in the long run, given restrictions on entry of dentists (or nonresponse of suppliers of dental education), is to increase output by using more inputs such as auxiliaries as well as by changing technology.

One further aspect differentiating these two types of supply subsidies is that the nature of the supply shift will differ. The HPEA program is equivalent to subsidizing new firms into the industry. These dentists will therefore have excess capacity in which to expand their supply of services over time; hence the new supply curve would be more elastic under this situation than when existing dentists hire more auxiliaries. In the latter case, the supply elasticity could be increased if auxiliaries were permitted to undertake more tasks. These restrictions are perhaps the constraining factor in the size of the dental "firm."

An additional assumption was that the supply of auxiliary training facilities would respond to increased demand. According to data presented in Chapter 4, the supply response of this sector has been very large and rapid. Last, the analysis treated auxiliaries as a homogeneous employee. In reality the different types of auxiliaries presumably have different productivities, and hence wages, and would possibly require different amounts of capital and equipment.

The policy alternatives examined up to this point have been on the supply side. The effect of an increase in supply is to lower the price of dental care and increase its use. The beneficiaries of such policies are those persons using dental care. Shifts in the supply of dental care will therefore presumably benefit those families in the middle and upper income levels, since dental care is income elastic and the decrease in price as a result of such supply programs is very slight. If the objective underlying such programs as the HPEA was one of equity — that is, to increase the amount of dental care to those with low incomes — then a subsidy program that directed its funds to those with low incomes would achieve this purpose at a lower cost than either a demand or supply subsidy to all persons. The HPEA program acts as a supply subsidy to *all* users of dental care, hence it would be comparable to a subsidy program to all the demanders of dental care.

A demand subsidy to just those with low incomes could be in the form of subsidized dental insurance; a supply subsidy for the purpose of benefiting just the low income families might be to provide forgiveness loans to students locating in poor areas upon graduation. However, under the HPEA, the loan forgiveness program is just a small part of the total federal subsidy benefiting the nonpoor. If supply subsidy programs are to be compared to demand subsidy programs for low income persons, then it should be realized that since the costs of education of all students are subsidized, the portion of supply subsidy dollars that end up increasing the supply for the poor is less than if the entire supply subsidy was provided directly as a demand subsidy for the particular population group to be assisted.

An analysis of the costs of alternative demand type subsidies is provided in Chapter 6. In that chapter a simulation program was developed to enable us to examine several demand subsidy programs together with more population characteristics than could be undertaken with the econometric model in its current form.

Summary and Conclusions

An econometric model of the dental sector was constructed in order to be able to evaluate policies and to make predictions for 1975. Theoretically the model was specified as having several levels; first was the market for dental care services, in which the measure of services is the patient visit. The second level was the market for dental manpower, with the demand for this manpower being derived from the demand for dental visits. The last level was the market for dental manpower training facilities, with the supply side of this market being considered as the primary constraint on the supply of dentists.

Because of the lack of data it was not possible to estimate the various markets in the detail we would have liked. The supply of visits was estimated as a function of both the price of a visit and of dentists per thousand population. The demand for visits was related to both price and income. We would have liked to have included additional variables such as the prices of inputs in the supply equation, and other demand variables such as age, education, and fluoridation in the demand equation. From the estimated supply and demand equations the reduced forms were calculated showing the equilibrium values of price and visits per thousand population. The supply of dentists was estimated as being determined by the supply of dental graduates (which is in turn determined by the number of dental school places), the existing supply of dentists, and losses from this supply through deaths and retirements.

The econometric model was used in three ways: the first was to forecast dental prices, utilization, total dental expenditures and dentists' incomes. Even without any subsidized national insurance plan for dental care, prices for dental care are expected to increase from 1970 to 1975 by 25-30 percent. Although visits per thousand population are also expected to increase, their increase is expected to be half as large as the increase in prices. Dental expenditures are expected to increase by 50-60 percent over this period and dentists' incomes by about 40-50 percent.

A comparison was then made between the ratio technique and the econometric model. It was shown that even with a constant dentist-population ratio, prices will still increase by 25-30 percent. More importantly, the ratio technique has a number of disadvantages when compared to the econometric model; the model is able to forecast the effects of a so-called gap in the dentist-population ratio in terms of increased prices and lower visit rates. The ratio technique does not provide any measures to indicate the importance of different sized gaps. Further, the model, by predicting visits rather than dentists as the measure of dental services, suggests alternative methods by which the demand for visits or the supply of visits may be increased. The supply of dentists is viewed as only one of several inputs into the production of dental visits. Thus implicit in these two methods is a difference in the approaches for achieving policy goals — which is the second use to which the model was put.

Because requirements based upon a ratio technique center on the number of dentists, proposed policies usually relate to increasing the supply of dentists through increasing dental school capacity. The econometric model, however, indicates that utilization can be affected by many factors on both the demand and supply side, and that there are also alternatives for increasing the supply of visits other than increasing the number of dentists.

In this regard a simulation analysis of the HPEA program was undertaken in order to show what its effects have been since it started. Forecasts of these effects were made through 1975. An analysis was then made to determine whether it would have been less costly to achieve the same increase in supply as provided under the HPEA program by increasing the use of auxiliaries. Assuming the proper functioning of the markets for auxiliaries and auxiliary training facilities, this latter program could have achieved the same goal more quickly and at a much lower cost. The econometric model can thus be used as a tool for the policy maker to compare alternative policies for achieving a common goal in terms of their effects on prices, utilization, and expenditures. The selection of a particular policy can be made on more objective grounds and with more information regarding its consequences.

The last use which the econometric model illustrated was a sensitivity analysis to determine on which areas of the model additional research would be most worthwhile. This analysis is presented in Appendix 5B. The importance, particularly for national dental insurance programs, of the accuracy of estimates of price elasticity of demand and the effect of having an increase in the supply of dentists was demonstrated.

While the results based on the econometric model should be considered as tentative due to the unavailability of some data, the several applications in which the model has been used should illustrate the usefulness of further research in this area. The increased information for forecasting and policy analysis resulting from a more detailed and more accurate model would certainly be worth the necessary costs of developing such an improved model.

Appendix 5A. Summary of Equations and Key to Variables

Equations

(1a) $\quad D_{VTH} = 1302.40 - 258.97 P_V + 1.22 Y$

(2a) $\quad S_{VTH} = -804.20 + 66.32 P_V + 3535.10 DTH$

(1b) $\quad \text{Log } D_{VTH} = -1.15139 - 1.43 \text{ Log } P_V + 1.71 \text{ Log } Y$

(2b) $\quad \text{Log } S_{VTH} = 3.24701 + .29 \text{ Log } P_V + 1.08 \text{ Log DTH}$

(3) $\quad DTH = DTH_{-1} + \Delta DTH$

(4) $\quad \Delta DTH = GTH - RTH$

(5) $\quad RTH = .02 DTH_{-1}$

(6) $\quad GTH = ETH_{-4} - PTH_{\Sigma 4}$

(7) $\quad PTH_{\Sigma 4} = .10 ETH_{-4}$

(8) $\quad ETH = STH$

(9) $\quad STH = STH_{-1} + NSTH$

(10) $\quad SNTH = \dfrac{SUB + MATCH}{\$308,000} + \dfrac{POP}{1,000}$

(11a) $\quad PV = 6.48 + .004 Y - 10.87 DTH$

(12a) $\quad VTH = -374.70 + .25 Y + 2814.37 DTH$

(11b) $\quad \text{Log } P_V = -2.55721 + .99 \text{ Log } Y - .63 DTH$

(12b) $\quad \text{Log VTH} = 2.50541 + .29 \text{ Log } Y + .90 \text{ Log DTH}$

(13) $\quad \text{Ln VPD} = 1.446 + .466 \text{ Ln AUX} + .777 \text{ Ln HRD} + .254 \text{ Ln CHR}$

Key to Variables

D_{VTH} = demand for dental visits per 1000 population

S_{VTH} = supply of dental visits per 1000 population

Y = per capita personal income

P_V = price per dental visit (calculated as $\dfrac{\text{mean annual gross income of dentists}}{\text{mean annual patient visits/dentist}}$)

DTH = dentists per 1000 population

STH = dental school spaces per 1000 population

NSTH = additions to dental school spaces per 1000 population

SUB = construction subsidy funds

MATCH = matching construction funds

POP = civilian population

ETH = first-year dental school students per 1000 population

GTH = dental school graduates per 1000 population
PTH = dental school dropouts per 1000 population
DTH = change in stock of dentists per 1000 population
RTH = dentists dying or retiring per 1000 population
VPD = annual patient visits per dentist
AUX = number of full-time auxiliaries employed by a dentist
HRD = number of annual hours worked by a dentist
CHR = number of chairs in the office

Appendix 5B.
A Sensitivity Analysis
of the Dental Model

The third use of an econometric model of the dental sector is to conduct sensitivity analysis. Confidence in the econometric model for both forecasting and policy analysis depends upon the accuracy of each of the coefficients in the model. Econometric research attempts to measure the effects of each of the factors believed to influence demand and supply of dental care. A change in any one of these coefficients will have different effects on the outcomes of the model; a large change in one coefficient may have minimal effects on the outcomes of the model, whereas a small change in another coefficient may cause large changes in the price and utilization of dental care.

Increased accuracy as to their true effects for those coefficients that can have large changes on price and utilization is desired. Research, therefore, should be directed to developing better estimates for these factors. Sensitivity analysis measures the relative size of the effects of price and utilization of dental care with respect to changes in the values of each of the coefficients in the model. The sensitivity analysis for the dental model was undertaken using the reduced forms in logarithms. This is because the coefficient of the log of an independent variable is its elasticity on the dependent variable. The demand and supply equations were:

$$\text{Log } D_{VTh} = -1.15139 - 1.43 \text{ Log } P_V + 1.71 \text{ Log } Y$$

$$\text{Log } S_{VTh} = +3.24701 + .29 \text{ Log } P_V + 1.08 \text{ Log } DTh$$

The reduced forms therefore were:

$$\text{Log } P_V = \frac{-(3.24701 + 1.15139)}{(.29 + 1.43)} + \frac{1.71}{(.29 + 1.43)} \text{ Log } Y - \frac{1.08}{(.29 + 1.43)} \text{ Log } DTh$$

$$\text{Log } VTh = \frac{3.24701 \,(1.43) - 1.15139 \,(.29)}{(.29 + 1.43)} + \frac{1.71 \,(.29)}{(.29 + 1.43)} \text{ Log } Y + \frac{1.08 \,(1.43)}{(.29 + 1.43)} \text{ Log } DTh$$

These reduced forms were not completely solved through in order to be able to observe the specific coefficients from the demand and supply equations.

If we want to observe how sensitive the price and quantity of dental care is to

171

changes in income we can examine that portion of the reduced forms that comprise the income effect, namely:

$$\text{Log } P_V = \frac{1.71}{(.29 + 1.43)} \text{ Log } Y$$

$$\text{Log } V_{Th} = \frac{1.71 \, (.29)}{(.29 + 1.43)} \text{ Log } Y$$

By referring back to the demand and supply equations, we observe that the income effect on P_V and V_{Th} is related to the price elasticity of supply (.29), the price elasticity of demand (−1.43), and the income elasticity of demand (1.71). If income was to increase by 10 percent what would be the effect on P_V and V_{Th}?

$$\text{Log } P_V = \frac{1.71}{(.29 + 1.43)} = \frac{1.71}{1.72} = .99 \text{ x } (10 \text{ percent increase in income})$$

$$\text{Log } V_{Th} = \frac{1.71 \, (.29)}{(.29 + 1.43)} = \frac{.49}{1.72} = .29 \text{ x } (10 \text{ percent increase in income})$$

With a 10 percent increase in income, therefore, prices would increase by an equivalent amount, 9.9 percent; while visits would only increase by 2.9 percent.

If, however, the price elasticity of supply was .5 instead of 2.9 how would this change the effect of an increase in income? In this case P_V would increase by 8.7 percent and V_{Th} would increase by 4.4 percent. The larger the price elasticity of supply, the smaller will be the increase in dental prices and the larger will be the increase in utilization. For example, if instead of .29 price elasticity of supply was 1.00, then P_V would increase by 7.0 percent and V_{Th} also by 7.0 percent, with a 10 percent increase in incomes. The consequences of changes in any of these coefficients are such that they can have important effects on total expenditures as well as total visits.

A sensitivity analysis was made of changes in each of the following coefficients: price elasticity of supply, price elasticity of demand, income elasticity, and elasticity of dentists per thousand population on supply. These results are summarized in Table 5B. The first column in this table indicates which of the above elasticities were unchanged. The second column indicates the new value, the third column shows which independent variable is increased by 10 percent, i.e., either income or dentists per thousand, and the last five columns show the percent changes in price, visits per thousand, total visits, total dental expenditures, and dentists incomes as a result of that 10 percent change in the independent variable.

The results of the sensitivity analysis can be summarized briefly. The smaller the price elasticity of demand, the greater will be the percent increase in price with a given percent increase in income (examples 1, 2, and 3). Large price

Table 5B. Sensitivity Analysis of the Dental Model

Case	Elasticity	Value	Ind. Var.	Percent Change In:				
				PV	VTH	TV	TE	DDSY
1	Demand(Price)	−1.43	Y	+ 9.9	+ 2.9	+ 2.9	+13.1	+13.1
2	Demand(Price)	−1.00	Y	+13.3	+ 3.8	+ 3.8	+17.6	+17.6
3	Demand(Price)	−0.66	Y	+18.0	+ 5.2	+ 5.2	+24.1	+24.1
4	Demand(Price)	−1.43	DTH	− 6.3	+ 9.0	+ 9.0	+ 2.1	− 7.2
5	Demand(Price)	−1.00	DTH	− 8.4	+ 8.4	+ 8.4	− 0.8	− 9.8
6	Demand(Price)	−0.66	DTH	−11.4	+ 7.5	+ 7.5	− 4.8	−13.5
7	Demand(Income)	1.71	Y	+ 9.9	+ 2.9	+ 2.9	+13.1	+13.1
8	Demand(Income)	1.20	Y	+ 7.0	+ 2.0	+ 2.0	+ 9.1	+ 9.1
9	Demand(Income)	1.71	DTH	− 6.3	+ 9.0	+ 9.0	+ 2.1	− 7.2
10	Demand(Income)	1.20	DTH	− 6.3	+ 9.0	+ 9.0	+ 2.1	− 7.2
11	Supply (Price)	0.29	Y	+ 9.9	+ 2.9	+ 2.9	+13.1	+13.1
12	Supply(Price)	0.50	Y	+ 8.7	+ 4.4	+ 4.4	+13.5	+13.5
13	Supply(Price)	1.00	Y	+ 7.0	+ 7.0	+ 7.0	+14.5	+14.5
14	Supply(Price)	0.29	DTH	− 6.3	+ 9.0	+ 9.0	+ 2.1	− 7.2
15	Supply(Price)	0.50	DTH	− 5.6	+ 8.0	+ 8.0	+ 2.0	− 7.3
16	Supply(Price)	1.00	DTH	− 4.4	+ 6.4	+ 6.4	+ 1.7	− 7.6
17	Supply(DTH)	1.08	DTH	− 6.3	+ 9.0	+ 9.0	+ 2.1	− 7.2
18	Supply(DTH)	1.50	DTH	− 8.7	+12.5	+12.5	+ 2.7	− 6.6
19	Supply(DTH)	1.08	Y	+ 9.9	+ 2.9	+ 2.9	+13.1	+13.1
20	Supply(DTH)	1.50	Y	+ 9.9	+ 2.9	+ 2.9	+13.1	+13.1

increases would also result in large increases in expenditures and dentists' incomes. Further, the smaller the price elasticity of demand, the greater will be the *decrease* in price with an increase in the stock of dentists (examples, 4, 5, and 6).

Changes in the estimate of income elasticity have little effect on the dependent variables when there is a change in the number of dentists (examples 9 and 10). With an increase in incomes, a larger estimate of income elasticity will result in increases in all the dependent variables but their increases will be less than for changes in price elasticity of demand (examples 7 and 8).

Increased estimates of price elasticity of supply have greater impact on the number of visits than on the price of dental care when there is an increase in demand for care (examples 11, 12, and 13). An increase in the coefficient of the number of dentists will of course have large effects on the supply of visits. If the coefficient of DTh was larger, then a given increase in the number of dentists will have a much larger effect on supply than if it were not so large. To the extent that restrictive practices decrease the size of this coefficient, its effects in terms of smaller supplies and higher prices can be observed.

The importance of these elasticity estimates can be seen when we consider the possible effects of a national insurance program for dental care under different assumptions of the price elasticity of demand. Depending on which elasticity estimate is used, the expenditures of such a program could be twice as much as expected. It would thus certainly be worthwhile to undertake research in order to havè a more accurate estimate of price elasticity (probably by income level) before any such program was undertaken.

The Role of Government in the Financing and Provision of Dental Services

The role of the government in the financing or in the operation of the market place is controversial, whether in health or nonhealth areas. This controversy regarding the role of the government is a result of two factors, never explicitly separated: (1) differences in values regarding what people would like to see occur, and (2) differences in opinion regarding the effect of a particular policy, namely, the effects of a particular policy on various population groups as to who will be better off than before and who will be worse off. It would be immodest to think that a single chapter could so clarify issues as to get rid of this controversy over the role of government with respect to the field of dental care; a more modest and attainable goal would be to separate the controversy into areas that result from differences in value judgments and those that result from differences in analysis or in empirical evidence. By so doing it will be possible to decide whether certain programs and policies really do achieve the goals they were intended to achieve and, further, to determine what are the "costs" of different goals or values. Only by having such information is it possible to decide whether alternative policies should be used, and whether some goals are more desirable than others because of their lower costs.

The purpose of this section is to provide a framework for the role of government in dental care, and in this manner to separate questions of analysis and empirical differences from those relating to differences in values. We will also attempt to indicate the most efficient way of achieving various values or objectives in dental care.

An Economic Framework for Government Intervention

There are certain economic problems that each society must solve, such as how much of a particular good or service should be produced, how should it be produced, how should it be distributed, and how do we allow for growth and change to occur in that sector. Within any society the decision making may take place through the market (voluntary exchange) or nonmarket (government) or a combination of both. An important philosophical question for society concerns the extent to which these economic problems should be handled through a competitive market process or left to government agencies.

Price theory, a major branch of economics, is concerned with how these economic problems are solved in a competitive market system; subject to some qualifications to be discussed below, a competitive market solves these problems

175

in as good a way, if not better, than any other alternative system, and should therefore be relied upon.

The basic economic problems of how much dental care and of what type, how best to produce it, who should receive it, and how to incorporate change in this sector, when decided within a competitive market framework in the dental sector, would result in the following approach toward solving these economic problems. The determinants of demand for dental care would influence how much and what type of dental services people were willing to buy; their distribution would also be left up to those with the greatest demands for such services. How "best" to produce such services would be determined by dentists attempting to produce such services subject to certain budgetary constraints facing them; change and innovation would be incorporated into the market as they are developed and present improved productivity or quality.

If these decisions were all made in a nonmarket context by a government agency, the performance of the two systems could be compared if the criteria used for comparison were similar. The criteria used in analyzing competitive systems involve efficiency on both the supply and demand side: is the care produced at minimum cost for a given level of quality; are consumers allowed to express their differing valuations of such care; do the different valuations which are placed on dental care by consumers also reflect the cost of producing it? Generally, persons favoring a nonmarket system for decision making may accept the criteria on the supply side (efficiency in production) but they rarely agree with the values implicit in the demand criteria — that people have different demands for dental care and place a different valuation on receiving it.

Under a market organized system people would not all be willing to spend the same amount of their budget on such care, or buy (and use) as much of it as someone would like them to. Persons favoring a market system for solving the basic economic questions of how much, how "best," etc., must implicitly accept these values. Unless the criteria involve efficiency in consumption as well as production, comparisons between market and nonmarket systems are not likely to be very fruitful.

Even a sector organized on the principles of a competitive market may occasionally be consistent with certain forms of government intervention. Government intervention, or nonmarket decision making, in a competitive market can be justified for the following reasons:

Redistribution or Equity. The belief that persons who have insufficient resources to purchase the desired amount of a market's product or services should be aided. The criteria used to finance the government's role in this case would be based on ability to pay.

Market Imperfections. That the competitive market, for various reasons to be discussed, does not operate efficiently. The criteria to be used in financing programs for correcting such inefficiencies would relate potential benefits to costs, and not ability to pay.

The reasons for government intervention suggest different roles for the government. It becomes necessary therefore to discuss these reasons in greater depth to determine what the legitimate roles are for government, and whether resultant government actions perform as expected. To be meaningful, the discussion of these possible reasons for government intervention assumes that these reasons can be separately handled. In this way it is possible to discuss the most efficient way of achieving each of the above objectives separately, e.g., equity, without the compromise and inefficiency of handling them jointly.

Market Imperfections and External Effects

Competitive markets might not function properly because of the disparity between how they actually function and how the theoretically "perfectly competitive" market is supposed to function. Further, even if these markets functioned as they theoretically should, with no imperfections, they may still not operate in an efficient manner because of "external effects." Therefore, each of these causes for nonmarket decision making, and the resulting proposed remedies, will be discussed.

Externalities and Public Goods

In a "perfectly" operating competitive market, the consumers and the providers, each acting to maximize their utility or their profits, will determine the quantity and quality of (in this case) dental care and how it should be produced. Efficiency in both consumption and production will result. If, however, there are external effects in either the production or consumption of oral health services, then an efficient solution will not occur. Externalities in consumption result if a person undertakes an action that affects others in the community; these external effects can either be favorable or unfavorable. Similarly, if a producer undertakes some action that affects others either favorably or unfavorably, these effects are also called externalities. The basic concept of externalities is that there is an interdependence of effects resulting from the actions of a consumer or producer and that the affected consumers or producers change their allocation decisions as a result of these external effects.

Because of these positive and negative external effects in both consumption and production, either too little or too much of a product or service will be provided. For example, if a factory pollutes a stream as part of the process of producing a product, then the costs for producing that product are understated; they do not include the costs of cleaning up the stream. Since the costs of that product are lower, its price is lower, hence more of it will be produced than if the costs of producing it reflected all the costs of production. In this instance the social costs (consisting of both the private costs of production and the costs of cleaning up the stream) exceed the private costs alone.

Alternatively, the private benefits that accrue to one person as a result of his fluoridating the community's water supply are less than the social benefits of his doing so, since others also benefit from his action, e.g., the other consumers have fewer caries, hence change the allocation of their expenditures. In this case the social benefits (consisting of both the private and external benefits) exceed just the private benefits as produced by the private market alone. In order to produce an optimal level of output, these external costs and benefits must be considered together with the private costs and benefits. Hence nonmarket (government action) decision making is required.

When just a few individuals are involved, they can get together and voluntarily agree upon a method of compensation and the optimal allocation of resources to produce the service. However, when large numbers of persons are involved then it becomes more difficult to make voluntary arrangements satisfactory to all concerned. Group decision making then, which is nonmarket in the sense that individuals are required to abide by the decisions of others (e.g., a government agency which may represent the group), is required in order to determine what the proper level of output should be and the compensation required.

It is when the allocation decisions of the indirectly affected consumers or producers are affected by external benefits or costs (through their utility or production functions) that compensation is required in order to achieve an optimal level of output. If the indirect consumers or producers are not affected "at the margin" by the external effects − i.e., there is no change in their allocation process − then their well-being (or income) may be affected but not their allocation process. Nonmarket decision making in order to achieve an optimal level of output is required when consumers' and producers' allocation decisions are affected at the margin.

Methods of compensation for external effects involve a system of taxes or subsidies based not upon ability to pay but on who benefits or who imposes additional costs on other persons. If compensation was not imposed, voluntary compensation might not be forthcoming. There are several forms of collective action available. In addition to a system of taxes and subsidies, the government could impose regulations, such as ordinances on the level of air or water pollution; or it could clean up such pollution itself, or subsidize others to do so. If either of these alternative governmental approaches is used, the external effects may be corrected but the level of output which was either excessive or insufficient would not be changed as a result of these administrative actions. This is because the private decisions are still made according to the private costs and benefits. Hence an optimal level of output would not be attained by such administrative actions.

Nonmarket decision making for other than external effects, such as for redistributing income, requires a different role of government and of method of compensation. For redistributive policies, the system of taxes and subsidies would be based on ability to pay rather than in relation to the distribution of external effects. Therefore, one reason for distinguishing between these different roles of government is to be able to specify the appropriate financing mechanism that should be used in each case.

An extreme case of externalities in consumption is the instance of a "public good" such as the provision of national defense. Not only are there external benefits in consumption when such a good is provided, but it is also impossible to exclude anyone from participating in those benefits. In the case of a public good, the amount that is required to satisfy the needs of one person is also sufficient to satisfy the requirements of all others, and they cannot be excluded from receiving those benefits. This contrasts to a purely "private" good, such as food, where the individual purchasing it receives all the benefits. The inability to exclude anyone from benefiting is what distinguishes a public from a private good – not whether the government or an individual finances it or produces it.[1]

Important questions regarding the dental sector are whether there are externalities in the production and consumption of oral health services; where they occur; and how they can be measured. The technique used in nonmarket decision making in this area is referred to as "cost-benefit analysis." Cost-benefit analysis is an attempt to measure benefits, including external benefits, from a program and relate this to the costs of achieving these benefits. This is generally easier to discuss than to achieve. The estimation of costs are usually more precise than the measurement of benefits. When there is no measure of the value people place on something (such as how much they would be willing to pay for a service) then how does one go about estimating the benefits they would receive from that service? The measurement of benefits in the health field has often been an estimate of the discounted future earnings of a person whose productivity would be entirely or partially lost if it were not for the particular program. This is grossly inaccurate. Some persons might be willing to spend much more than the discounted earnings of a child in order to prevent their child from becoming ill or crippled.

There are no easy methods of evaluating the benefits people may receive from programs that have external effects.[2] Simple measures, such as the effect on productivity, hence earnings, resulting from a program, may be either too high or too low. A major problem in nonmarket decision making is specifying the benefits from externalities and measuring them. Some persons when discussing the health field have simply stated that it is obvious that external benefits exist in the provision of *personal* medical care services, usually giving examples from the field of public health, and then gone on to justify all sorts of government programs using a financing principle based on ability to pay, which further confuses the issues.

The application of cost-benefit analysis to the dental sector, with its concomitant approach toward financing those benefits, requires an explicit discussion of external benefits. In what follows, I will provide my concept of where the externalities exist in dental care and where they are nonexistent. The reader should be aware that we are now in an area where there is no unanimity among economists working in the field of health; this discussion should serve as a point of departure for further analysis in an attempt to make explicit what has heretofore simply been assumed to exist.

Fluoridated water supplies and research on oral health are, I believe, clear examples of goods that have external benefits. If a community's water supply is fluoridated, then the benefits cannot be denied to anyone in that community. Cost-benefit analyses of whether or not to fluoridate the water supply would therefore be appropriate and have in fact been conducted. The case of external benefits with fluoridation may not be as obvious as it appears. A large number of persons in a community may believe that there are actually negative external effects from having fluoridated water supplies. If this were the case then instead of taxing them to help support the fluoridation program, it may be necessary to subsidize them in order to compensate them for being worse off. Alternatively, since topical fluorides and fluoride pills are available, even though they may be less effective and more costly than simply fluoridating the community's water supplies, this may be seen as a method of internalizing any externalities.

Similarly, the benefits (findings) from basic research are also generally freely available. If a charge (greater than the cost of disseminating such information) had to be paid in order for a person to ascertain the findings of such research, then this would be economically inefficient, since the opportunity cost of its availability is zero. The great uncertainty involved in research (and the uninsurability of such risks) together with the inability to appropriate the gains means that the amount of basic research that will be undertaken without a subsidy will be smaller than the socially optimum amount.

Cost-benefit analyses of how much should go toward dental research would also be appropriate, but unfortunately they are more difficult to conduct. Support of research to develop methodologies and estimates of the optimal level of dental research expenditures would therefore be desirable. The existence of externalities however does not mean that all such services should be financed nationally. With respect to fluoridation, since the benefits are local, the financing mechanism should also be local. With dental research, however, the benefits are nationwide, hence the financing mechanism should be national in scope.

Except for fluoridation and dental research, I find it difficult to find support for the contention that there are external benefits in other areas of the dental sector, particularly with regard to dental education. External effects with regard to redistribution of dental services might exist if those with greater access or ability to purchase dental care believed that those less fortunate than they should also have some level of care or access to it. In this case if one wealthy person provides for redistribution then other persons also receive the benefit of seeing those with less dental care receive more. An external benefit has thus been created and should be compensated by having the other persons receiving this benefit also contribute toward it.

The government, acting as the agent in this example of nonmarket decision making, would collect taxes from those receiving the increase in benefits and subsidize the recipients, according to the preferences of the donors. The objective of this program is to maximize the utility of the donors, rather than that of the recipients. This type of program may result in providing dental services in a form or manner that is more acceptable to the donors than the recipients. It is important to specify whose preferences are being satisfied as a result of a subsidy program. This is discussed in greater detail in the section on redistribution where it is assumed that the recipient's preferences are to be maximized.

There is a great concern that dental education, to include both the schools and the students, should be heavily subsidized. This subsidy may be rationalized by its proponents in terms of either externalities or for reasons of income redistribution. In addition to the externalities argument, there may be other market imperfections that would suggest some form of subsidization. Imperfections in the capital market would reduce demand below optimal levels because a loan made to an individual to finance his education in a nonslave state with no other security to offer other than his future earnings is a less attractive investment than a loan on tangible property where the collection costs would also be lower. There is an additional imperfection in the market for risk bearing. Because the return to an investment in a professional education is somewhat risky and if one were to insure against this risk there would be a problem of moral hazard, i.e., the insured might "take a job that is not monetarily remunerative after graduation. . ." A possible solution to such market imperfections are not subsidies to the educational institutions, but rather a national loan program with an income contingent repayment plan.[3]

In this section the justification for such a subsidy in terms of externalities will be discussed; in the section on redistribution this form of subsidy will also be considered. The belief in externalities of dental education implies that the supply of dental manpower should be larger than would be provided under a perfectly operating market. In order to achieve a greater number of dentists than would be forthcoming in a perfectly operating market, potential dentists would have to be subsidized to enter the profession. This subsidy would compensate them for the lower rate of return resulting from lower incomes, as a result of lower prices from having a larger supply.

One reason for wanting a larger supply of dentists might be a desire for excess capacity so that anyone requiring a dentist would always be able to see one. However, increasing supply would presumably result in lower prices, hence, increased visits, and not necessarily in unused available dentist time. A person needing dental services would still have to pay for them. Therefore, if the desire for excess capacity was to insure that a person requiring a dentist always be able to receive the necessary care, then the subsidy should be given to the person needing the services or only to those dentists willing to provide emergency care at a free or reduced price.

Similarly, the idea that an increased supply of dentists should be available through a subsidy so that "they'll be there if you need them" again suggests that the subsidy should either go to the consumer or the dentist that locates in an area where they are most "needed," i.e., where the variance in demand for dental care is greatest (not where there is the greatest demand for care) and in those places where there is chronic excess demand because it may be in a relatively unattractive location. Subsidizing all dentists (or dental students) in this latter case would be inefficient because they may locate in the wrong places.

Thus even if there were some merit (external benefit) to having more dentists than would be provided by the private market, the subsidy should be provided to either the prospective patient or a particular group of dentists — not all consumers, all dentists or students, nor the dental school. However, it is not clear that there is an external benefit to having more dentists. Emergency requirements in dental care are not large, relative to the total demand for dental care, and the costs of delay in such a system are probably small. Therefore it seems that the external benefits that would accrue to everyone as a result of decreased waiting time to see a dentist are much less than in other areas of medical care and are probably not the primary reasons for subsidies to dental schools, students, and auxiliary personnel.

Another reason used for subsidizing education is the notion that everyone benefits from having people educated, therefore there are external benefits to all.

Economists have made some progress in recent years in identifying and measuring the external effects of elementary and secondary education, but the externalities of higher education, if any, are much more subtle and elusive . . . Unless, however, the external benefits to society can be measured and valued, even if only crudely, the case for subsidies to higher education remains weak.[4]

If the professional education is purely private, in that it increases the economic productivity of a person, and that person can capture that higher productivity through higher earnings, he has an incentive to invest in the necessary educational requirements. This return would be sufficient to cause a substantial amount of education to be produced and sold in a private market; government subsidy of this education would not be required in order to produce an optimal quantity.

If there are external benefits (as defined earlier) to dental education beyond the purely private benefits, then it should be subsidized. However, since it is not intuitively obvious that there are such external effects to a dental education, then the supporters of such subsidies should offer more evidence as to those effects.

Market Imperfections

The performance of a market, measured in terms of prices and quantities of services and the degree of innovation, is related to a number of factors, each of which will have certain effects on performance. Some of the more important theoretical characteristics of a competitive market which cause the market to perform in an optimal fashion are:

1. Many buyers and sellers, no one of which is large enough to have influence on the price of the product or service sold nor on the wages (or prices) paid for its inputs

2. No restrictions on entry either into the industry or into the area where the firm wishes to locate, or on tasks performed by any one person

3. Consumers, knowledgable regarding the prices of different products they buy, their respective quality and of the benefits of purchasing the particular good or service

4. Producers, also knowledgable regarding the prices they must pay for factors of production, and of the contribution to output of different quantities of particular personnel

The fact that markets in the real world differ from the theoretical ideal with respect to one or more of the above assumptions is not sufficient cause for entirely dispensing with a market approach for production and distribution of products and services. The reason being that the therapy may be more painful (or more damaging) than the disease. Each of these prerequisites for an optimal market has an effect on performance if it is not achieved (or achieved to a lesser degree). It would be useful to determine the extent to which these characteristics deviate from their theoretical ideal, what the effect of this is likely to be in terms of performance, and the suggested role for government when these market imperfections exist.

The number and size of firms. One cause of market imperfection is if the least-cost size of firm is so large in relation to the market it serves that it becomes feasible to have a single firm serve the entire market. Such a case, known as declining long-run average costs, precludes competition from a market since only one firm is viable. The role of government in a case of natural monopoly is either to regulate it (as with public utilities) or to operate it itself. Examples of natural monopolies in the provision of dental services are nonexistent. As discussed in Chapter 3, The Supply of Dental Care, there appear to be some economies with increased size but that these economies are reached at a relatively small scale. Therefore, in any urban area we would expect to find a larger number of dental firms. Although the number varies depending upon size of city, region of the country, etc., it appears that the economies of scale occur in an operation small enough to insure that the theoretical condition of a competitive market is not unduly violated. Thus it would appear that this does not present a role for the government, such as decreasing the concentration of an industry with regard to the number and size of dental firms.

The level of knowledge among consumers and producers of dental services. To the extent that the consumer is knowledgable regarding the prices he must pay for dental care, of the quality of the care he buys, and of prices and quality between different dentists, then the consumer will choose to spend his limited funds in the most utilitarian way possible. He may decide he would prefer paying a lower price and receiving a lower quality of care, given his budget. Recognizing that people place different values on receiving dental care, and that they have limited incomes, they might not spend their funds on particular needs in similar fashions. However, unless a group explicitly decides that other people ought to spend their money as the group feels they ought to (which would be inconsistent with a market, or "voluntary" approach to decision making), then one is forced to accept the manner in which those funds are spent.

However, consumers are not very knowledgable of the benefits of dental care and oral hygiene, nor do they have much information of prevailing prices and differing qualities in the market for dental services. Their choices as to the quantity and quality of the care they buy is also imperfect, thus imperfection in the market for dental services exists with regard to consumer knowledge. This lack of consumer knowledge on dental prices and quality, however, is not accidental; it appears to be a deliberate policy to keep the consumer as ignorant as possible with respect to information that will enable him to choose on the basis of price and quality. (There are a few limited examples where such information is available.) This same policy exists in other aspects of the health field, such as with physician and hospital care. The professional reasons for not providing the consumer with such information are that it would either be "unethical" to have price competition among dentists, or that the consumer would not be able to judge differing levels of quality even if criteria could be developed.

An additional reason why consumers of dental services might be ignorant of the prices and quality of different providers is that there is a cost associated with consumers gaining such knowledge. Given the level of expenditures on dental care as a proportion of income, a consumer might be unwilling to spend the necessary resources, including the time and effort, to become "knowledgable." The cost of gaining such information, however, is increased if the providers are inhibited from publicizing it.

Regardless of the reasons and value judgments for not making this information available, it should be possible to analyze the consequences of such action in terms of market performance. First, the less information available to the consumer for making choices means that he must either invest his own time in gathering the data or that he might make a poorer choice than if it were available. Second, the inability of the consumer to make price and quality comparisons might serve to maintain prices at a higher level than they would be otherwise. Last, the inability to have prices related to quality differentials among providers prevents calculations by the consumer on the marginal value to him of higher quality.

The inability to relate prices to quality also has allocative effects: the return on higher quality training cannot be priced in the market and is thus determined by other factors to be discussed below. By not publicizing information on quality of care as practiced by individual dentists, the dental profession has attempted to maintain the quality of dental care through the use of "process" measures. This approach toward quality will be discussed in the section below on restrictions in the dental market.

Producer Knowledge and Information

The level of information available to the producers of dental services appears to be relatively high. For example, the American Dental Association provides information on various locations so that migrating or graduating dentists have more information on factors affecting their locational decisions. There have also been numerous studies indicating the increased value to dentists of using auxiliary personnel. Perhaps implicit in the discussion of producer knowledge is the assumption that there is an incentive on their part to use information to become as efficient as possible in producing dental services, given the legal restrictions on how they can use certain inputs. To the extent that the necessary information is either not available to the producer or that the incentive is not very strong, then there will be "slack," i.e., the firm *could* produce more for a given budget than it currently does.

Although the level of producer information and the incentives toward efficiency could be increased, it is not obvious that this requires government intervention. Part of these functions (i.e., information) is currently being handled by various other groups, e.g., the professional associations. (If the government became a large purchaser of dental services, then it might wish to be concerned with the efficiency with which dental services are produced. It is possible that the level of information and incentives are related to the level of competition in the market for dental services. The more restricted the competition, the less incentive there is for the provider to be efficient. In order to determine the degree of competition, and whether there is a need for government intervention, it is necessary to examine the barriers to entry and other restrictions in the dental sector.

Mobility and Entry Restrictions

Perhaps the largest deviation from the theoretical model of a competitive dental care market occurs in the area of restrictions. There are three types of restrictions to consider: barriers to entry into dental schools and the dental profession; restrictions on mobility between locations where a dentist may practice; and restrictions on tasks that auxiliaries may perform. The supposed objective of such restrictions are to insure high quality of dental care. However, their effect — for example, entry barriers to dental schools, — is to limit the number of persons who can become dentists, cause higher dental incomes, a smaller supply of dental services, and higher prices for services than would exist without such restrictions. (Restrictions on the tasks that auxiliaries perform might in fact have necessitated a larger supply of dentists than if greater delegation of tasks were permitted.)

Important questions are whether the benefits of restrictions are worth the cost of achieving them; whether there are alternative ways of achieving their benefits at lower costs; and, who benefits from restrictions. The answer to the last question might provide an indication as to the real motivation behind restrictions as compared to the stated reasons. The stated purpose of many of the restrictions in the field of medical care is that they are in the public interest — they increase quality! The consumer of dental care is unaware of the quality of care practiced by his dentist; the costs of poor quality of care may be quite high (depending on the illness and the treatment); therefore it becomes necessary to regulate the quality of care provided. The method generally used to insure high quality of care is to specify educational requirements in accredited educational institutions, to limit the dental tasks performed by less "qualified" persons, and to require a licensing exam.

The prime emphasis of quality control is on the process of achieving quality — educational requirements and restriction of tasks. Once a person has been licensed as a dentist there are few or no controls on the quality of care that he renders. If the purpose of much of these restrictions is to achieve high quality of dental care, then what are some alternatives?

The Quality Question. Let us divide the quality question into two parts: the quality of care received by persons going to dentists, and the overall quality of dental care in the remainder of the population. Both these aspects of quality are related; in fact they are inversely related since the longer it takes to train a dentist, the fewer dentists there are, hence fewer persons see dentists.

If we accept the level of dental care received by the entire population as one measure of the quality of dental care of the current system, then this level of care should be determined by weighting the number who receive dental care and those who do not receive any care. Some societies would score much higher on this measure of quality since their cutoff point for those who can practice dentistry is lower than in the U.S., hence more persons can receive some dental care.[5] The astronomical figures of unmet dental needs in this country are testimony to the quality measure we have accepted; we concentrate only on those who already receive care. This is the inevitable result of placing standards for quality in the hands of the professionals themselves.

Basing licensure on educational requirements and a one-time licensing exam tells us nothing about the actual quality of care practiced by the dentist or whether he keeps up in his field. According to one study, though not in dentistry, licensing is no indication of the quality of the service actually rendered; and if quality is to be assured in a market where the consumer is ignorant of the service he purchases, then there must be continual surveillance of the service performed by the providers.[6]

The regulation of quality of dental care for those who receive it by emphasizing the dentist's qualifications rather than his continual performance appears to be a less than optimal quality control system. Its effect, whether intended or not, is to lengthen the time required to become a dentist, decrease the number of dentists, and does not, in fact, monitor the actual quality of care practiced. Assuming that the objective were to raise or to monitor the quality of care practiced, then a system that measured quality both directly and frequently would be more accurate than one which did not.[7] Further, a system that explicitly recognized different levels of quality of dental care that are practiced would provide more information to consumers than one which had as its goal the establishment of a minimum level with no recognition of higher levels of quality.

It might be argued that the costs of a system for regulating quality on an outcome basis would be too great; however, if such a system was to be instituted then scarce resources currently devoted to producing quality inputs could be released if they were not really effective. Further, although such information is costly to produce, it has a value in that people would be willing to pay for information to improve their choices.

Concentration on the outcomes of quality. Concentrating on technical excellence of any unit or service, a filling, a crown, etc., rather than on its input requirements would have a number of additional advantages. There might be greater incentives to restructure curriculums in dental schools if it could be demonstrated that such educational changes led to measurable increases in quality; or it might show that it is possible to produce the same level of quality with shorter periods of training. If it was possible to calculate the increase in quality as a result of increased training, then this additional cost of higher quality can be examined to determine its worth in terms of what people are willing to pay or in the additional numbers of dentists that could have been produced. We would not expect quality of dental care to become uniformly low. Since there would be a demand for different levels of quality, different levels of quality would be supplied, as occurs with other goods and services in the economy.

Educational requirements. The emphasis on long educational requirements as a means of controlling quality is increasingly being used by dental auxiliaries. Economists, perhaps because of their basic cynicism, have developed alternative hypotheses regarding increased educational requirements for various professions.

Economists would hypothesize that any profession likes to control the number of persons in that profession, because it affects their incomes.[8] Therefore we would expect various methods be used to limit entry: requiring a long dental education in order to become a dentist, limiting the number of dental schools, placing additional barriers in the way of those who wish to enter the supply (e.g., impose an educational requirement on foreign dental graduates), and include elements in licensing exams that are unrelated to quality.[9] This hypothesis would suggest that the emphasis on quality will be on the criteria for entering the profession rather than on the care practiced by the profession.

If the emphasis was on the care practiced then the profession would find it difficult to justify supply restrictions. An interesting hypothesis regarding increased specialization in medicine is given by C. M. Lindsay: raising education requirements, such as taking boards in various specialties, even in general practice will have the effect of decreasing the number of physicians, since it lowers their rate of return by increasing their opportunity costs — the foregone income for additional years spent in school. That is, the longer one is in school, the less lifetime there is to earn a living, thereby reducing lifetime earnings and the rate of return for entering that profession.

If physicians with higher levels of training were permitted to publicize them, then they would be able to receive higher prices for their services, which might offset their greater loss in foregone earnings. However, if increased training requirements are viewed merely as a device to restrict supply and to benefit the *existing* supply of physicians, then they would not want any information available for consumers to judge the different levels of quality. Lindsay concludes that if periodic licensing examinations for physicians was instituted, it would become obvious that there are different levels of quality in medicine; rather than eliminating those physicians at the lower end, the profession would merely acknowledge their existence. Recognition of different quality levels of physician care would also eliminate the incentive for present physicians to favor increased levels of training for entering physicians, because this additional training could then be differentiated.[10]

An economic view of restrictions. As a means of decreasing supply, restrictions on the tasks not permitted to auxiliaries would be a supply limiting measure. As demand for dental care continues to increase, we would expect more dentists to be using more auxiliaries, since it would increase their incomes. We would further expect that auxiliaries (acting not unlike other professions) would attempt to raise educational requirements for entrants to their profession and also propose a licensing requirement. These proposals would undoubtedly limit their supply, hence increase the wage that dentists must pay. The dental professional would thus be up against a similar method of raising quality in one of the factor inputs they must employ. Further, there will be, as in the medical profession, suggestions for having auxiliaries (or a better trained auxiliary) perform more tasks that are currently in the domain of the dentist. Since such auxiliaries represent a substitute for the dentist's services, we would suppose that the dental profession would favor such a change only if the auxiliaries were under the *control* of a dentist. In this way a possible substitute becomes a complementary factor in the production of dental services.

The economist's view of restrictions may be cynical; however, it provides a set of hypotheses that are testable. That is, restrictions in the field of dental care will be promulgated as being in the public interest by the particular profession proposing them only if, in the economist's view, it has the effect of raising that profession's income. In the economist's view, restrictions represent a market imperfection. However, the role of the government has been to sanction and even to legalize them. If the market for dental care is to perform in a more efficient manner, i.e., produce a greater supply of care at a lower cost, then ways must be sought to handle the goals of quality, which restrictions purport to do, in a more direct manner and to rely more on these techniques and less on restrictions.[11]

Income Redistribution: Government Financing of Personal Dental Services

Two reasons were suggested as justifications for government intervention in the market for dental services. The first was because of imperfections in the market as a result of externalities; the criteria used would be that those persons receiving the benefits, e.g., from fluoridation or dental research, should bear the costs. The second reason for government intervention would be if there are market imperfections as a result, for example, of restrictions resulting in monopoly power.

A third reason would be if it were decided that there were persons with insufficient resources to purchase goods and services (or dental care) through the market and that subsidies should be provided in order to enable them to increase their consumption of these goods and services. In this latter case it is assumed that the market mechanism for distributing and producing goods and services is adequate but that income transfers are required in order to make that distribution more equitable. The financing mechanism to be employed in this latter case would be based on "ability to pay," namely, those receiving the benefits do not pay all or any of the costs and that the beneficiaries be of relatively lower incomes.

An evaluation of income redistribution policies would determine who the beneficiaries are of the various programs that are explicitly or implicitly aimed at a redistribution of resources, and whether the desired group of beneficiaries receive a net "benefit" after the various subsidies and methods to finance those subsidies are considered. The net benefits going to each income class should be calculated, and if the objective is to achieve a redistribution, presumably the largest net benefits should go to the lowest income classes. What often occurs in those programs that may be considered as redistributive, as in subsidies to higher education, is that they actually provide greater net benefits to those in the higher income classes.[12]

Redistribution programs should also be compared to other possible redistribution programs in order to determine which ones provide the greatest net benefit per dollar spent to a particular income class. Assuming that funds for redistribution are scarce, the allocation that maximizes the desired redistribution would be preferable to any other set of redistribution programs. In order to make these nonmarket decisions, however, information on net benefits by beneficiary groups for different programs are necessary.

Before discussing different methods of redistribution as applied to dental care, the objectives and implicit values of such programs should be considered more fully. Comparison of programs that differ either with respect to objectives or values would not be useful in determining how to achieve a given objective most efficiently. It is for this reason that the role of government in dental care was separated: financing nonpersonal dental services (that is, market imperfections caused by externalities), and this section on financing personal dental services.

Cash vs. In-Kind Subsidies

One objective of redistribution programs is to maximize the utility of the recipients. If we assume that low income persons have many needs for which they have insufficient resources, and if it was deemed desirable to assist them in meeting these needs, the best judge of how these subsidies should be spent would be the recipients themselves. If this were the objective of the program then subsidies should be given in cash to the recipients. Any other form of redistribution does not achieve the desired objective as efficiently as does a cash subsidy; they would be better off receiving the cash equivalent of the in-kind subsidy.[13] An implicit value judgment by the donors in such cash subsidy programs is that the recipient is the best judge of his needs and that he would not squander away these subsidies.

Another form of redistribution is to provide in-kind subsidies. In-kind programs provide subsidies for particular goods and services, e.g., housing, Medicare, etc. The method used to provide such subsidies may be in the form of tax credits, subsidized rents, public housing, free clinics, and so forth. The purpose of in-kind subsidies is for the recipient group to increase their consumption of a particular good or service. The value judgments of the donors underlying in-kind subsidies are that increased consumption of this particular good or services is more important in their opinion than other goods that the recipient would buy if he were just given cash. There may be an underlying fear on the part of the donors (or proponents of the subsidy) that the recipients are not capable of making rational choices.

The proponents of in-kind subsidies, which are the predominate form of subsidy in this country, may also have another motivation. They may be the producers of the particular good or service being proposed for the subsidy and this would, in effect, increase their demand, hence their incomes. Regardless of whether the proponents are financially affected by the subsidy program or whether they simply think that the recipients require this particular good more than others, the objective of in-kind subsidy programs is to maximize the preferences of the *donors*. The recipients will in all likelihood receive a net benefit, but it would not be as large as the benefit from the cash equivalent of the in-kind subsidy.

The objectives of income redistribution programs therefore must be explicitly stated if evaluations are to be made of alternative programs to achieve that objective.

. . .it is not clear whether taxpayers are concerned with the recipient's income, consumption, or utility. If income is the focus, it would suggest that society (apart from recipients) is concerned only that all individuals have some opportunity for minimum consumption. In this case, direct money transfers are probably the preferred activity, although it is legitimate to consider investments which generate equivalent income streams for the recipients as alternatives. If consumption is the focus, transfers in kind are indicated, such as provision of housing, food, clothing or whatever are the important items of consumption from the donor's point of view. If the utility of the recipient is the focus, the mechanism of transfer itself must be included in the evaluation.[14]

Alternative Methods of Providing In-Kind Subsidies

Decisions regarding cash or in-kind subsidies are outside the scope of this book; they are made at a broader level than the dental sector. However, once these decisions are made and it is decided to provide in-kind (dental services) subsidies, then additional decisions must be made: what are the alternative means by which they can be provided; who are the beneficiaries of each of these alternative subsidies; which programs offer the greatest net benefits (for a given budget) to the desired group of beneficiaries?

An in-kind subsidy for dental care can be given directly, by purchasing dental insurance for the beneficiary population, or indirectly, by subsidizing the supply side of the dental sector. In the latter case the price is lowered by increasing the supply. There are also alternative mechanisms within each of these demand and supply type methods of subsidizing the consumption of dental care services. Ideally it would be desirable to show the consequences of choosing between demand and supply type subsidies, between different methods within each, and for different beneficiary groups under each of the above alternatives. Perhaps a word should be said concerning the method used to raise the funds under any financing program. A tax program that relies on a proportional or progressive tax will generate more dollars from the higher income groups than from those with lower incomes. A number of proposals for financing health insurance, however, rely on a regressive form of taxation; namely, a percentage tax on a certain part of ones income. A Social Security tax will result in a higher *percentage* tax on a lower income person than will a program that is funded from general income tax revenues. Since the data for making such comparisons in the dental sector do not currently exist, what follows will be only an attempt to answer these questions, to the extent that the limited data permit.

A direct subsidy for dental care to a particular population group will result in an increase in the amount of care demanded by those recipients. The amount by which the quantity demanded will increase will depend upon the responsiveness of the recipient's consumption of care to price reductions (price elasticity of demand) and the extent to which the price is lowered to them. An increase in the quantity of care demanded by this group will result in an increase in the total demand for dental care and with it an increase in the price of dental care. The extent of this increase in price will depend upon the size of the increase in care demanded, how elastic or inelastic supply is, i.e., how responsive supply is in the short run to higher prices of dental care and the method used for reimbursement. Some methods of reimbursement will provide less of an incentive for dentists to raise prices — or at least by as much — than others. These increased prices will in turn serve to reduce the amount of care demanded by others not similarly subsidized.

Again, the amount by which the quantity demanded will be reduced by these other groups will depend on how responsive their use is to changes in the price they must pay (price elasticity). Under a demand subsidy therefore, the beneficiaries will be those receiving the subsidy, and the dentists, since both the price and demand for dental services will increase. Those bearing the costs of this program will be the nonsubsidized demanders of dental care, who face higher prices for care, and the taxpayers.

The advantage of a demand subsidy is that it goes directly to the beneficiaries who are to be assisted. Its difficulties are the probable higher prices of care that will result, particularly if the increase in quantity demanded is large and supply cannot be expanded quickly, i.e., elasticity of supply is low. An indirect subsidy to increase the consumption of dental care for particular beneficiary groups would attempt to increase the supply of dental care; for example, providing scholarship assistance so as to increase the numbers of health manpower. Important to any supply subsidy is the responsiveness of supply to such subsidies. The effect of such subsidies will be to lower prices of dental care (or more realistically, they would not rise as rapidly as they might) and to increase utilization.

The extent to which price will be lowered and utilization will be increased will depend upon the size of the increase in supply and the price elasticity of demand. The beneficiaries of supply subsidies will be the users of dental services, since the prices to them will be lower. Those bearing the burden of such supply subsidies will be the taxpayers, and existing dentists whose incomes might have been slightly higher if the increase in supply were achieved by increasing the number of dentists.

There are alternative methods that could be used on the supply side; subsidies could also be provided to achieve an increase in dental auxiliaries. It would require fewer years to produce more auxiliaries and the beneficiaries of such a program, in addition to the ones mentioned above, would also be the dentists; they would be able to hire more of this input at a lower wage than they would have paid previously. We would presume that dentists would favor such a program while existing auxiliaries would not be enthusiastic since it would tend to dampen their wages. We would expect that auxiliaries would propose longer educational requirements as well as licensing (as other professions have done) as the number of auxiliaries began to increase, in order to keep their incomes up.

The difficulties with supply subsidies are several. First, their effects are indirect; they might not result in an increase in the consumption of dental care by those for whom it would be most desirable. Second, policies to increase supply take a long time; at a minimum it requires six years to increase the number of dentists assuming that the facilities and personnel exist to train them. Third, the beneficiaries of supply subsidies are generally higher income families, not only because they use more dental services but also because the students receiving the scholarships come from families with higher incomes. Further, any subsidy of a specific input on the supply side lowers its price, causing a greater substitution toward use of that input in the production process. This would be a less efficient way of increasing the supply than providing unrestricted supply subsidies to firms so that they can decide on the optimum combination of resources, if the markets were operating freely.

This brings us to the last difficulty with supply subsidies. We believe they are used to mask the inefficiencies that result from restrictions on the supply side. If there are barriers to entry into the profession — not only in the number of students admitted but also in artificially maintained educational requirements — these cause a shortage of dentists, who in turn will receive a persistently excess rate of return.

The solutions to such shortages in the health field is generally to pour sufficient quantities of funds into the existing educational market in order to achieve an increase in supply. This is a very expensive method of achieving relatively small increases in supply, given the objectives of high quality by the educational institutions, their nonprofit nature, and the lack of incentives to increase output in order to receive government subsidies. The costs of restrictive practices in dentistry (and in other areas of medical care) are not as visible if there is an increase in supply as a result of a massive infusion of subsidies.

Nationally Subsidized Insurance for Dental Care

Assuming that society decides to provide an in-kind dental subsidy, what are the likely goals of such a subsidy, what are the alternative strategies for achieving such goals, and what is it likely to cost?

Proposals for government financing of dental care as discussed above can be limited to subsidizing the demand for dental care, subsidizing the supply, or subsidizing some combination of both. In order to simplify the matter, the demand and the supply aspects will be separated and government financing with respect to the demand side will be discussed here. Earlier, supply subsidies to dental education were discussed. However, since estimates of the likely supply will affect the future prices of dental care, different assumptions regarding supply must be incorporated into the discussion of the costs of different government financing programs.

There could be several goals or value judgments with respect to subsidizing the demand for dental care. One such set of values might be that everyone should receive a minimum amount of dental care. Another set of values might propose that everyone should have equal access to dental care, while still a third set of values would suggest that dental care should be free to all. Each of these set of values represents a different demand for subsidization of dental care services.[15]

If it was decided that everyone should be able to afford a minimum quantity of dental care, this goal could be achieved by making dental care free to all, or merely subsidizing those whose consumption is below the minimum. The costs of achieving each of these alternatives varies greatly, as will be shown below. It would be less costly to achieve the set of values favoring minimum provision if dental care was subsidized for just those below the minimum. Therefore making dental care free to all would be an inefficient way of achieving the goal of minimum provision.

If, on the other hand, the goal were equal access to dental care for all then this could also be achieved in alternative ways; dental care could be free to all or the consumption of dental care could be subsidized for certain population groups. Since there are differences in attitudes toward seeking dental care, free care for all would still not lead to equal consumption; equal access will also not lead to equal consumption, but it will eliminate those differences in dental consumption that are a result of economic constraints. If equal consumption or for that matter, minimum consumption was actually desired, then this set of values might actually suggest *paying* those below the minimum (or with unequal consumption) to receive dental care. The payment might be in cash or it might be in the form of subsidies for travel to the dentist, and so forth.

The most efficient way of achieving equal access would also involve a subsidy that varied according to the person's consumption of dental care, rather than by making it free to all. A free dental service would involve unnecessarily large costs for achieving the objective of equal access. If the supply of dental care was relatively "inelastic," i.e., it required proportionately higher and higher prices to achieve a given increase in supply of services, then the costs of achieving any of the above set of values, by making dental care free, become increasingly more expensive.

The above discussion can be demonstrated graphically as follows: assume there are three income classes, i.e., high, middle, and low income, and that their demand curves are respectively HI, MI, and LI, as shown in Figure 6-1. The total demand for dental care would be the sum of these three demands and is shown as HABC. If the price of dental care was OP_1, and the supply of care was assumed to be completely elastic (for simplicity), then the consumption of low income persons would be QL, the middle income persons would consume QM, and high income persons QH. The aggregate consumption of dental care would be QT. The use of dental care would therefore be greatest among the higher income families and lowest among those with least income. It is assumed, again for purposes of simplicity in exposition, that demand for dental care is only a function of price and income and that there are no income effects, and further that the three groups are of similar size.

If it was decided to subsidize the use of dental care so that everyone received a minimum quantity, e.g., Qx, then this could be achieved by lowering the price (subsidization) to those with lowest income to OP_2 (this could be achieved, for example, by using a co-pay of varying amounts, e.g., 20 percent). The cost of this policy would be the amount by which price is lowered multiplied by the quantity of visits used by that group, shown by the area OQX times $P_1 P_2$. Aggregate demand for dental care would increase from QT to QA (which is equal to Qx − QL).

The alternative to this approach of increasing everyone's consumption of dental care until it is at least Qx is to lower the price of dental care to all, by either giving everyone a subsidy or just making it free to all. The effect of this would be to increase the aggregate demand for dental care to OC, since everyone in each income category would consume OI (which is equal to the sum of I − Qx and I − QH). The cost of this would be OC multiplied by OP_1, which is much greater than the more limited subsidy program to achieve the same desired objective.

If instead of minimum provision the goal was to achieve equal access, then the analysis would be quite similar. In order to have those with lower income consume QH of dental care, which is what the high income families use, then the price of low income families should be lowered to OP_3, while for those with middle incomes the price should only be lowered to OP_4. In this way everyone will be consuming QH of dental care (assuming, for purposes of exposition, that the only differences between groups is an economic constraint). Aggregate demand in this case will increase more, to OQG. The cost of the variable subsidy program will be the proportion of the price that is subsidized multiplied by the quantity

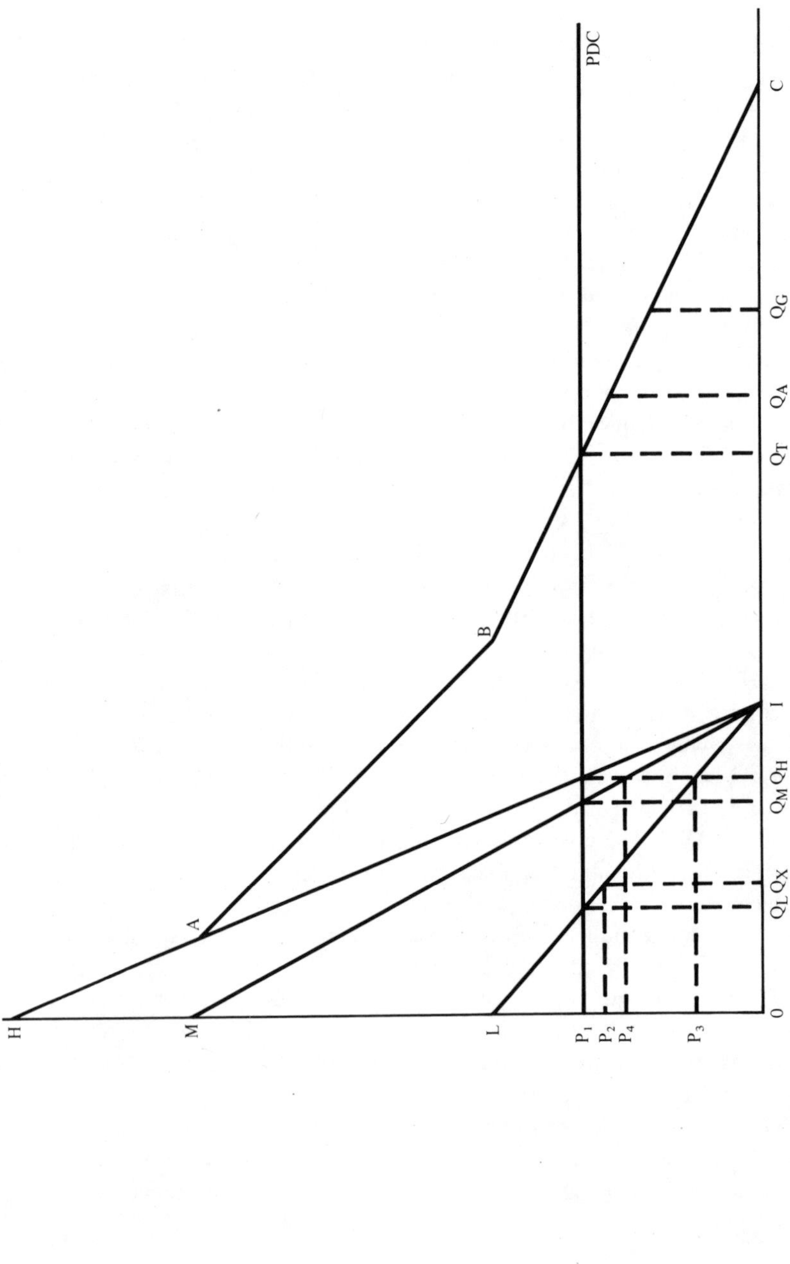

Figure 6-1. The Demand for Dental Care by High, Middle, and Low Income Families

of care consumed. Although this objective of equal access is more costly to achieve than the goal of minimum provision, they are still both less costly than free provision.

If, as is true in the real world, the price of dental care is not constant, i.e., that supply is not perfectly elastic, then the costs of each program will be even higher. Unless supply was perfectly inelastic with respect to price, the more inelastic it is, the greater will be the "inefficiency" of free provision (i.e., higher cost for a given objective) in achieving each set of values. Also, the greater the price elasticity of demand for dental care, the greater will be the inefficiency of free provision. As shown earlier, the demand for dental care is not completely price inelastic.

To summarize this discussion, therefore, if it is desired to achieve either of the set of values implied by minimum provision or equal access, then it would be least costly to do this with a subsidy that varied according to income rather than an equal subsidy to all or a free dental service.

In the next section an attempt is made to estimate the "costs" of such alternative policies for subsidizing the purchase of dental care.

Estimates of Alternative National Insurance
Plans for Dental Care

In an attempt to make more explicit the choices with respect to financing dental care, some forecasts were made of the probable utilization, costs, and effects on different population groups of alternative national insurance plans for dental care. If the costs of such alternative plans could be estimated, our ability to choose between them would be improved; therefore a simulation analysis of possible alternative plans was conducted.

Forecasts of the effects of alternative dental insurance plans were built upon three basic considerations: first, what features will be incorporated into such plans with regard to coverage, controls, and population groups; second, what is likely to be the effect of limits or controls (or lack of them) on use; third, what is likely to be the price of dental care, since, in order to determine expenditures under alternative programs one must multiply utilization by some expected price. Each of these aspects will be briefly discussed before presenting the estimates under each set of assumptions.

Possible Features of Alternative National Insurance
Plans for Dental Care

The basic features that may be incorporated into different insurance plans relate to the existence and size of deductibles and coinsurance and what population groups are to be included, either with the same coverage or with differing deductibles and coinsurance. It is possible to consider other limits such as treatment specific coverage, however because of the limited data available, any estimates of this feature, or similar ones, would be top hypothetical to be useful. The possible choices that were considered were:

1. No deductible, no coinsurance — i.e., full coverage

2. A $20 deductible and a $40 deductible

3. A 20 percent and 40 percent coinsurance feature

4. Combinations of deductibles and coinsurance together

5. Variable coinsurance according to family income

For those persons in the lowest income categories there would not be any coinsurance, while for progressively higher income levels the coinsurance would increase until it was 100 percent at the highest income levels.

    An analysis of the effects of each of these possible features was conducted for six age groups within each of six income classifications. Two time periods were also used for this simulation, 1970 and 1975. The initial data on visits and population for each of these age-income categories are presented in the tables of Appendix 6.

The Effect of Various Insurance Features
on Dental Utilization

An aspect that may drastically affect any forecasts of the utilization (hence cost) of a national insurance plan is the effect that lowering the price of the service will have on the recipients. In most instances the forecasts of utilization under national programs both in this country and in others such as Great Britain have been inaccurate because the effect of lowered prices on use turned out to be different — usually higher — than was anticipated. The effect of prices on utilization, "price elasticity," was discussed earlier in the section on demand. In those analyses an attempt was made to estimate the price elasticity of demand for dental care. The empirical estimate of price elasticity appeared to be approximately minus one, meaning if price of dental care was raised or lowered by 10 percent, there would be an equivalent 10 percent change in usage (in the opposite direction from the price change). Ideally it would be useful to know the responsiveness of increased use to decreased prices by income level; however, it was not possible to derive such estimates with currently available data, however, one could infer the effects of different price elasticities for each income group by examining the simulation that assumed different price elasticities for all groups.

    Since the assumption regarding price elasticity of demand is so central to the use and cost of different insurance plans, several different estimates were used in the simulations. One estimate was that price elasticity was -1.00. Another estimate assumed that it was $-.66$. This latter estimate implies that if the price of dental care were reduced by 10 percent then use of dental services would increase by only 6.6 percent. In the former case, i.e., price elasticity was -1.00, it was assumed that dental use would increase by 10 percent, equivalent to the percentage change in price.

The large differences in expenditures that resulted when different estimates of price elasticity were used strongly suggest that this would be a worthwhile area for future research if we are to be able to forecast more accurately the cost of different insurance plans.

The Price of Dental Care
Under National Dental Insurance

Estimates of the cost of the different insurance plans must translate the utilization that is likely to occur into expenditures. In order to do this, some estimate of the future price of dental care is required. It is likely that the price paid for dental care will be affected by the method of reimbursement and the degree of controls employed in monitoring payments. However, a prime determinant of dental prices is, as was discussed earlier, the size of the increased demand and the responsiveness of supply to such demand increases. The likely price after insurance is instituted is another aspect which has consistently led to inaccurate forecasts of government programs; the costs of both Parts A and B under Medicare were seriously underestimated before such programs were instituted. (Forecasts of dental prices under differing conditions would, therefore, be another worthwhile area for research.) Small differences in the estimates of future prices can lead to large differences, as will be shown, in the expenditures of alternative programs. If such information were fully known beforehand, it might affect our choices with regard to either coverage, population groups included, method of reimbursement used, or possible policies with respect to the supply of dental care.

In Chapter 5, dealing with forecasting, an attempt was made to estimate the likely increase in dental prices as a result of increased demands for care. It was shown that from 1970-1975 price increases without any new insurance program are likely to be quite large (25-30 percent), given the relative unresponsiveness of the supply side of the dental sector. Therefore, in making estimates of the likely cost of different insurance programs, several estimates of future prices are used. The higher estimates are more likely, the greater the comprehensiveness of the coverage (fewer controls or limits), the larger the population to be included under the insurance plans, and the further into the future that such forecasts are made. It should be noted that the estimates of demand and prices that are likely to prevail in 1975 are likely to be understated. This is because many of the other determinants of dental utilization that are likely to change, such as attitudes, have been held constant.

Two sets of simulations were conducted, for 1970 and 1975. The reason for using 1970 was to show what the consequences would have been had different types of policies been instituted. Since the population estimates are fairly accurate, the differences in the costs of the different programs can be attributed to program differences or to differences in prices and price elasticities. When program costs are forecast to 1975, then the accuracy of the population estimates have a bearing on the program costs as well. For 1975 only one set of population estimates have been used; however, it would be desirable to estimate the program costs, hence demands for service, under different assumptions about the size and age-income distribution of the population. In this way a range of estimates for each set of possible programs could be developed and costed out. (This approach could easily have been done but it would have required a great many additional tables in order to present these results here.)

For ease in calculating the consequences of a large number of possible alternatives within a national dental insurance plan, a simple simulation program was developed which generated for each change in coverage, price of dental care, and estimate of price elasticity, the following set of outputs:

1. The new set of visit rates for each age group within each income classification

2. The total number of visits demanded within each age and income grouping

3. Expenditures per capita within each age and income grouping and then categorized by the amount that would be the federal portion (in dollars) and consumer expenditures per person

4. Total expenditures within each age and income grouping, and the amount of that which would be federal and consumer expenditures

5. A few summary statistics such as total visits, total expenditures, total federal, and total consumer expenditures

A more complete description of how the simulation model makes the above calculations and the input requirements for its operation is available upon request.

The results of the simulations are summarized in Tables 6-1 through 6-4. The following are some general comments regarding the effects of different features within a possible national dental insurance plan.

The most expensive dental insurance program would be one which provided for free access to dental care for everyone. If this unlikely event occurred then the estimates of what it would cost would be, at a *minimum*, 9.7 billion dollars a year. (Current expenditures on dental care, both private and government, are approximately 4.5 billion dollars.) With the limited supply of dental care available it is not clear that the low income persons would receive more care; and prices, if not controlled, certainly would increase greatly. In fact, if the supply of dental care under such a situation were to be rationed, then those persons

Table 6-1. Visits and Expenditures under Alternative National Health Insurance Plans (1970)

Price = $14.00 *Elasticity = −0.66*

Policies	D = $00. C = .00	D = $20. C = .00	D = $00. C = .20	D = $20. C = .20	D = $00. C = .40	D = $40. C = .00	D = $40. C = .40	D = $00. C = .00 .20 .40 .60 .80 1.00
Visits								
Total (1000's)	689,901.9	456,932.5	475,073.4	352,301.3	369,565.1	235,730.7	235,730.7	328,932.8
Per 1000 Pop.	3479.87	2304.77	2396.27	1779.18	1864.01	1189.03	1189.03	1659.14
Expenditures								
Consumer (1000's)	0.0	3,000,305.0	1,330,202.0	3,386,685.0	2,069,560.0	3,300,226.0	3,300,226.0	2,497,893.0
Federal (1000's)	9,658,623.0	3,396,747.0	5,320,814.0	1,545,530.0	3,104,342.0	0.0	0.0	2,107,161.0
Total (1000's)	9,658,623.0	6,397,052.0	6,651,023.0	4,932,216.0	5,173,906.0	3,300,226.0	3,300,226.0	4,605,054.0

Price = $14.00 *Elasticity = −1.00*

Policies	D = $00. C = .00	D = $20. C = .00	D = $00. C = .20	D = $20. C = .20	D = $00. C = .40	D = $40. C = .00	D = $40. C = .40	D = $00. C = .00 .20 .40 .60 .80 1.00
Visits								
Total (1000's)	1,448,699.0	759,013.2	694,671.7	430,404.0	457,234.4	226,276.1	226,276.1	421,564.2
Per 1000 Pop.	7307.25	3828.47	3505.44	2170.96	2306.29	1141.34	1141.34	2126.37
Expenditures								
Consumer (1000's)	0.0	2,929,881.0	1,945,075.0	3,594,032.0	2,560,506.0	3,167,866.0	3,167,866.0	2,657,628.0
Federal (1000's)	20,281,776.0	7,696,304.0	7,780,318.0	2,476,619.0	3,840,764.0	0.0	0.0	3,244,264.0
Total (1000's)	20,281,776.0	10,626,182.0	9,725,401.0	6,025,654.0	6,401,278.0	3,167,866.0	3,167,866.0	5,901,897.0

D = Deductible

C = Coinsurance rate, where .00 represents full coverage. For the graduated coinsurance rate policy, the income breaks are as follows: C=.00, $0-2999; C=.20, $3000-4999; C=.40, $5000-6999; C=.60, $7000-9999; C=.80, $10,000-14,999; C=1.00, $15,000+.

Table 6-2. Visits and Expenditures under Alternative National Health Insurance Plans (1970)

Price = $16.50   Elasticity = −0.66

Policies	D = $00. C = .00	D = $20. C = .00	D = $00. C = .20	D = $20. C = .20	D = $40. C = .00	D = $00. C = .40	D = $40. C = .40	D = $00. C = .00 .20 .40 .60 .80 1.00
Visits								
Total (1000's)	689,901.9	473,803.4	451,254.6	343,914.5	343,811.1	343,811.1	215,719.5	307,997.4
Per 1000 Pop.	3479.87	2389.87	2276.13	1734.71	1734.19	1734.19	1088.09	1553.54
Expenditures								
Consumer (1000's)	0.0	3,123,886.0	1,489,136.0	3,634,023.0	2,269,150.0	2,269,150.0	3,559,371.0	2,708,712.0
Federal (1000's)	11,383,377.0	4,693,872.0	5,956,552.0	2,040,564.0	3,403,726.0	3,403,726.0	0.0	2,373,241.0
Total (1000's)	11,383,377.0	7,817,756.0	7,445,698.0	5,674,590.0	5,672,883.0	5,672,883.0	3,559,371.0	5,081,958.0

Price = $16.50   Elasticity = −1.00

Policies	D = $00. C = .00	D = $20. C = .00	D = $00. C = .20	D = $20. C = .20	D = $40. C = .00	D = $00. C = .40	D = $40. C = .40	D = $00. C = .00 .20 .40 .60 .80 1.00
Visits								
Total (1000's)	1,448,699.0	806,544.0	635,699.7	410,559.5	196,819.6	407,560.6	196,819.6	385,721.5
Per 1000 Pop.	7307.25	4068.22	3206.47	2070.87	992.76	2055.74	992.76	1945.58
Expenditures								
Consumer (1000's)	0.0	2,973,267.0	2,097,703.0	3,733,454.0	3,247,518.0	2,689,891.0	3,247,518.0	2,752,363.0
Federal (1000's)	23,903,520.0	10,334,703.0	8,390,835.0	3,040,766.0	0.0	4,034,845.0	0.0	3,612,034.0
Total (1000's)	23,903,520.0	13,307,968.0	10,488,545.0	6,774,223.0	3,247,518.0	6,724,751.0	3,247,518.0	6,364,404.0

D = Deductible

C = Coinsurance rate, where .00 represents full coverage. For the graduated coinsurance rate policy, the income breaks are as follows: C=.00, $0-2999; C=.20, $3000-4999; C=.40, $5000-6999; C=.60, $7000-9999; C=.80, $10,000-14,999; C=1.00, $15,000+.

Table 6-3. Visits and Expenditures under Alternative National Health Insurance Plans (1975)

Price = $16.50   Elasticity = −0.66

Policies	D = $00. C = .00	D = $20. C = .00	D = $00. C = .20	D = $20. C = .20	D = $40. C = .00	D = $00. C = .40	D = $40. C = .40	D = $00. C = .00 .20 .40 .60 .80 1.00
Visits								
Total (1000's)	789,339.0	601,977.9	516,294.9	423,229.3	246,811.7	393,365.6	246,811.7	331,207.5
Per 1000 Pop.	3773.20	2877.58	2468.00	2023.12	1179.81	1880.37	1179.81	1583.24
Expenditures								
Consumer (1000's)	0.0	3,409,373.0	1,703,767.0	4,124,151.0	4,072,394.0	2,596,207.0	4,072,394.0	3,295,987.0
Federal (1000's)	13,024,094.0	6,523,264.0	6,815,088.0	2,859,129.0	0.0	3,894,315.0	0.0	2,168,934.0
Total (1000's)	13,024,094.0	9,932,636.0	8,518,864.0	6,983,282.0	4,072,394.0	6,490,532.0	4,072,394.0	5,464,923.0

Price = $16.50   Elasticity = −1.00

Policies	D = $00. C = .00	D = $20. C = .00	D = $00. C = .20	D = $20. C = .20	D = $40. C = .00	D = $00. C = .40	D = $40. C = .40	D = $00. C = .00 .20 .40 .60 .80 1.00
Visits								
Total (1000's)	1,657,504.0	1,080,785.0	727,290.2	525,118.7	225,187.7	466,303.4	225,187.7	399,435.9
Per 1000 Pop.	7923.21	5166.38	3476.60	2510.18	1076.44	2229.03	1076.44	1909.39
Expenditures								
Consumer (1000's)	0.0	3,276,420.0	2,400,051.0	4,354,023.0	3,715,593.0	3,077,597.0	3,715,593.0	3,258,960.0
Federal (1000's)	27,348,832.0	14,556,543.0	9,600,231.0	4,310,433.0	0.0	4,616,396.0	0.0	3,331,723.0
Total (1000's)	27,348,832.0	17,832,912.0	12,000,290.0	8,664,460.0	3,715,593.0	7,694,003.0	3,715,593.0	6,590,690.0

D = Deductible

C = Coinsurance rate, where .00 represents full coverage. For the graduated coinsurance rate policy, the income breaks are as follows: C=.00, $0-2999; C=.20, $3000-4999; C=.40, $5000-6999; C=.60, $7000-9999; C=.80, $10,000-14,999; C=1.00, $15,000+.

Table 6-4. Visits and Expenditures under Alternative National Health Insurance Plans (1975)

Price = $20.00 Elasticity = −0.66

Policies	D = $00. C = .00	D = $20. C = .00	D = $00. C = .20	D = $20. C = .20	D = $40. C = .00	D = $00. C = .40	D = $40. C = .40	D = $00. C = .00 .20 .40 .60 .80 1.00
Visits								
Total (1000's)	789,339.0	621,671.9	483,009.9	405,925.4	274,350.2	359,499.2	234,913.6	305,189.3
Per 1000 Pop.	3773.20	2971.72	2308.89	1940.41	1311.45	1718.48	1122.94	1458.87
Expenditures								
Consumer (1000's)	0.0	3,522,085.0	1,932,033.0	4,441,365.0	4,439,650.0	2,875,988.0	4,543,099.0	3,610,526.0
Federal (1000's)	15,786,782.0	8,911,356,0	7,728,155.0	3,677,142.0	1,047,359.1	4,313,989.0	155,174.9	2,493,258.0
Total (1000's)	15,786,782.0	12,433,441.0	9,660,198.0	8,118,411.0	5,487,008.0	7,189,987.0	4,698,274.0	6,103,788.0

Price = $20.00 Elasticity = −1.00

Policies	D = $00. C = .00	D = $20. C = .00	D = $00. C = .20	D = $20. C = .20	D = $40. C = .00	D = $00. C = .40	D = $40. C = .40	D = $00. C = .00 .20 .40 .60 .80 1.00
Visits								
Total (1000's)	1,647,504.0	1,066,836.0	650,034.0	465,021.1	190,545.4	404,796.4	190,545.4	358,067.7
Per 1000 Pop.	7923.21	5099.70	3107.30	2222.90	910.85	1935.01	910.85	1711.64
Expenditures								
Consumer (1000's)	0.0	3,314,800.0	2,600,129.0	4,511,920.0	3,810,912.0	3,238,367.0	3,810,912.0	3,369,859.0
Federal (1000's)	33,150,080.0	18,021,920.0	10,400,541.0	4,788,500.0	0.0	4,857,552.0	0.0	3,791,494.0
Total (1000's)	33,150,080.0	21,336,672.0	13,000,683.0	9,300,425.0	3,810,912.0	8,095,929.0	3,810,912.0	7,161,357.0

D = Deductible

C = Coinsurance rate, where .00 represents full coverage. For the graduated coinsurance rate policy, the income breaks are as follows: C=.00, $0-2999; C=.20, $3000-4999; C=.40, $5000-6999; C=.60, $7000-9999; C=.80, $10,000-14,999; C=1.00, $15,000+.

receiving care under a queueing system would be those who can afford (and are willing) to wait; these persons presumably would not be those with relatively low incomes. Thus a "free" dental care system, where queues result, also has "costs."

Since the probable cost of a program would be one factor influencing its feasibility, other possible national dental insurance plans would certainly include some controls both with regard to use and to the population groups covered. If deductibles are used to control costs then they are likely to exclude the low income families from any benefits. Currently low income families spend less on dental care than the likely size of a deductible. Therefore, if a plan had a high, say, of $40 per person deductible and after the deductible was paid additional care was free, then the prime beneficiaries (in addition to the dentists) would be those currently spending more than that amount and those expecting to. Those would be the higher income families. As can be seen in the tables, the imposition of deductibles reduces the size of the program in terms of federal expenditures, but it does not achieve the objective of increasing the utilization by the lower income users of dental care.

The use of a uniform coinsurance feature of say, 20 percent, would provide some benefits to everyone, including the low income families. However, the federal cost of such a program for 1970 would have been anywhere from five billion dollars (assuming the price only rises to $14 a visit and the price elasticity is −.66) to 8.39 billion dollars (assuming a price elasticity of −1.00 and a price per visit of $16.50). Instead of providing the same program benefits such as a flat coinsurance feature for all, to all income groups, fewer federal dollars would be required if the program concentrated on the lower income families.

A plan that had no deductible feature but an increasing copayment for families with higher incomes would provide maximum benefits to the lowest incomes and no benefits to those with the highest incomes; the federal expenditures under this type of program would have been approximately 2.1 billion dollars in 1970 (assuming a price elasticity of −.66 and a price per visit to all of $14). Total funds spent on dental care, federal and private, under this program would be 4.6 billion dollars. If we assume an elasticity of −1.00 and a price per visit of $16.50, then the federal expenditures would be 3.6 billion dollars and total expenditure would be 6.4 billion dollars.

As shown in Tables 6-1 to 6-4, the costs of all the various plans will increase in 1975, if for no other reason than that there will be an increase in population which, by increasing demand, is likely to cause an increase in the price of a dental visit. The forecasts of costs for 1975 are all similar in their relative magnitude for 1970, but the federal dollars involved for even the most minimal programs are expected to be much higher.

It is conceivable that some national dental insurance plans (even if price of a visit, price elasticity, and population size were unchanged) would be more expensive to begin with and would decrease in cost over time. Similarly, some plans that are very inexpensive to begin with will become more costly in the future. For example, if a national insurance plan for dental care included a high deductible after which the price of dental care was greatly reduced, then few persons would at present exceed the deductible limit. However, as incomes increase personal expenditures will begin to exceed the deductible provision (if it is not changed) hence the plan has the potential for being very costly for the insurer. Conversely, if a plan had a coinsurance provision that increased with increased family incomes, then as peoples' incomes increased over time fewer people would qualify for the lowest coinsurance categories while more of the population would move into those income classes with higher (or full) copay. Such a plan would, in addition to meeting the needs of the low income persons, gradually phase itself out over time.

It should be noted that the different estimates of price elasticity result in quite large differences in both federal and personal expenditures on dental care. If with a higher estimate of price elasticity the price of a visit remained the same – which is unlikely since with a sizeable increase in demand prices are likely to rise – then the magnitude, just for different estimates of price elasticity, is in the billions, depending again on the features selected for a dental insurance plan.

Further, the cost of any dental insurance plan, as well as the portion paid for by consumers, is affected by changes in the price of a dental visit. Holding constant the various features of a plan, as well as price elasticity, an increase in the price of a visit is likely to add hundreds of millions of dollars to the amount expended for dental care. This higher cost of any program, as a result of increased prices, indicates the return – the reduction in expenditures that could be achieved – if prices did not rise as rapidly.

Price controls are one method of limiting price rises; alternatives would be measures that increased supply, either of manpower within the existing structure of tasks or of changes in the job structure itself. The importance of such changes in supply become even more visible when the differences in expenditures as a result of such changes can be demonstrated.

The consequences of reducing the price of a service through the introduction of a dental insurance plan with similar benefits for persons of all income levels that is both income elastic and has some price elasticity is that the projected cost of such a program is likely to be larger than if there were no "moral hazard" involved. Further, if the program objective was to minimize the total program costs of increasing care to those with low incomes, then any dental insurance plan that does not do this directly will have much greater costs, and will be less efficient in achieving the desired objective.

Appendix 6A.
1970 Dental Visit Rates, By
Age and Family Income

Appendix 6A. 1970 Dental Visit Rates, by Age and Family Income

Age	\$0-2,999	\$3,000-4,999	\$5,000-6,999	\$7,000-9,999	\$10,000-14,999	\$15,000+
0 – 4	0.1	0.3	0.4	0.3	0.4	0.6
5 – 14	0.8	1.0	1.2	1.7	2.2	3.2
15 – 24	1.4	1.2	1.4	1.9	2.0	2.5
25 – 44	1.0	1.1	1.0	1.4	2.0	2.4
45 – 64	0.8	1.2	1.2	1.4	1.8	2.5
65+	0.6	1.0	1.3	1.7	1.3	2.6

(Family Income)

Source: Unpublished data from the U.S. National Health Survey.

Appendix 6B. 1970 Population (in 000's) by Age and Family Income

	Family Income					
Age	$0-2,999	$3,000-4,999	$5,000-6,999	$7,000-9,999	$10,000-14,999	$15,000+
2 – 4	1061	1274	1591	2440	2653	1591
5 – 14	4125	4951	6187	9489	10,317	6187
15 – 24	3957	4408	5419	8243	8914	5341
25 – 44	5557	5926	7209	10,909	11,756	7038
45 – 64	5784	5294	6173	9146	9717	5794
65+	6336	2970	2375	3366	2970	1782

total population 2 yrs. and over 198,255

Source: Dentistry in National Health Programs, Reports of the Special Committees, American Dental Association, October 1971, p. 42.

Appendix 6C. 1975 Population (in 000's) by Age and Family Income

Age	Family Income					
	$0-2,999	$3,000-4,999	$5,000-6,999	$7,000-9,999	$10,000-14,999	$15,000+
2 – 4	1014	1161	1275	1973	3132	3017
5 – 14	3470	3857	4242	6556	10,413	10,026
15 – 24	4001	4053	4403	6740	10,640	10,177
25 – 44	5691	5501	5932	9039	14,220	13,548
45 – 64	5471	4557	4794	7171	11,132	10,458
65+	5806	3440	2366	3656	3440	2795

total population 2 yrs. and over 209,196

Source: Dentistry in National Health Programs, Reports of the Special Committees, American Dental Association, October 1971, p. 43.

211

Appendix 6D.
Sample Output from Computer
Simulation Program

Appendix 6D. Sample Output from Computer Simulation Program.

Analysis of a $0.0 Deductible Dental Insurance Program, 1970

| Copay | 1.00 | 0.0 | 1.00 | 1.00 | 1.00 | 1.00 | 1.00 | 1.00 | 1.00 | 1.00 | 1.00 | 1.00 | 1.00 | 1.00 |
| | 1.00 | 1.00 | 1.00 | 1.00 | 1.00 | 1.00 | 1.00 | 1.00 | 1.00 | 1.00 | 1.00 | 1.00 | 1.00 | 1.00 |

Price per visit w/o insurance 12.20

Total price per visit with insurance 12.20

Elasticity −0.67

Family Income Age	Visit Rate	Total Visits	Total Expenditure per Capita	Consumer Expenditure per Capita	Federal Expenditure per Capita	Consumer Total Expenditure	Federal Total Expenditure	Total Expenditure
$0–2999								
0–4	0.10	106.1	1.22	1.22	0.0	1294.4	0.0	1294.4
5–14	4.05	16700.0	49.39	−0.0	49.39	0.0	203739.6	203739.6
15–24	1.40	5539.8	17.08	17.08	0.0	67585.4	0.0	67585.4
25–44	1.00	5557.0	12.20	12.20	0.0	67795.4	0.0	67795.4
45–64	0.80	4627.2	9.76	9.76	0.0	56451.8	0.0	56451.8
65+	0.60	3801.6	7.32	7.32	0.0	46379.5	0.0	46379.5
$3000–4999								
0–4	0.30	382.2	3.66	3.66	0.0	4662.8	0.0	4662.8
5–14	1.00	4951.0	12.20	12.20	0.0	60402.2	0.0	60402.2
15–24	1.20	5289.6	14.64	14.64	0.0	64533.1	0.0	64533.1
25–44	1.10	6518.6	13.42	13.42	0.0	79526.8	0.0	79526.8
45–64	1.20	6354.0	14.64	14.64	0.0	77518.7	0.0	77518.7
65+	1.00	2970.0	12.20	12.20	0.0	36234.0	0.0	36234.0
$5000–6999								
0–4	0.40	636.4	4.88	4.88	0.0	7764.1	0.0	7764.1
5–14	1.20	7424.4	14.64	14.64	0.0	90577.6	0.0	90577.6
15–24	1.40	7586.6	17.08	17.08	0.0	92556.3	0.0	92556.3
25–44	1.00	7209.0	12.20	12.20	0.0	87949.8	0.0	87949.8
45–64	1.20	7407.6	14.64	14.64	0.0	90372.6	0.0	90372.6
65+	1.30	3087.5	15.86	15.86	0.0	37667.4	0.0	37667.4

Sample Output from Computer Simulation Program (Continued)

Family Income Age	Visit Rate	Total Visits	Total Expenditure per Capita	Consumer Expenditure per Capita	Federal Expenditure per Capita	Consumer Total Expenditure	Federal Total Expenditure	Total Expenditure
$7000–9999								
0– 4	0.30	732.0	3.66	3.66	0.0	8930.4	0.0	8930.4
5–14	1.70	16131.3	20.74	20.74	0.0	196801.6	0.0	196801.6
15–24	1.90	15661.7	23.18	23.18	0.0	191072.5	0.0	191072.5
25–44	1.40	15272.6	17.08	17.08	0.0	186325.4	0.0	186325.4
45–64	1.40	12804.4	17.08	17.08	0.0	156213.4	0.0	156213.4
65+	1.70	5722.2	20.74	20.74	0.0	69810.8	0.0	69810.8
$10,000–14,999								
0– 4	0.40	1061.2	4.88	4.88	0.0	12946.6	0.0	12946.6
5–14	2.20	22697.4	26.84	26.84	0.0	276908.1	0.0	276908.1
15–24	2.00	17828.0	24.40	24.40	0.0	217501.5	0.0	217501.5
25–44	2.00	23512.0	24.40	24.40	0.0	286846.3	0.0	286846.3
45–64	1.80	17490.6	21.96	21.96	0.0	213385.1	0.0	213385.1
65+	1.30	3861.0	15.86	15.86	0.0	47104.1	0.0	47104.1
$15,000+								
0– 4	0.60	954.6	7.32	7.32	0.0	11646.1	0.0	11646.1
5–14	3.20	19798.4	39.04	39.04	0.0	241540.3	0.0	241540.3
15–24	2.50	13352.5	30.50	30.50	0.0	162900.4	0.0	162900.4
25–44	2.40	16891.2	29.28	29.28	0.0	206072.4	0.0	206072.4
45–64	2.50	14485.0	30.50	30.50	0.0	176716.9	0.0	176716.9
65+	2.60	4633.2	31.72	31.72	0.0	56525.0	0.0	56525.0
TOTALS		319037.2				3688506.0	203739.6	3892245.0

Analysis of a $0.0 Deductible Dental Insurance Program, 1975

Copay   1.00   0.0   1.00   1.00   1.00   1.00   1.00   1.00   1.00   1.00
            1.00   1.00   1.00   1.00   1.00   1.00   1.00   1.00   1.00   1.00

Price per visit w/o insurance   12.20

Total price per visit with insurance   16.50

Elasticity   −0.67

Family Income Age	Visit Rate	Total Visits	Total Expenditure per Capita	Consumer Expenditure per Capita	Federal Expenditure per Capita	Consumer Total Expenditure	Federal Total Expenditure	Total Expenditure
$0–2999								
0– 4	0.08	82.9	1.35	1.35	0.0	1367.8	0.0	1367.8
5–14	4.05	14048.2	66.80	–0.0	66.80	0.0	231795.6	231795.6
15–24	1.14	4579.4	18.89	18.89	0.0	75560.3	0.0	75560.3
25–44	0.82	4652.7	13.49	13.49	0.0	76769.0	0.0	76769.0
45–64	0.65	3578.2	10.79	10.79	0.0	59041.1	0.0	59041.1
65+	0.49	2848.0	8.09	8.09	0.0	46992.2	0.0	46992.2
$3000–4999								
0– 4	0.25	284.9	4.05	4.05	0.0	4698.4	0.0	4698.4
5–14	0.82	3153.3	13.49	13.49	0.0	52029.2	0.0	52029.2
15–24	0.98	3976.2	16.19	16.19	0.0	65607.8	0.0	65607.8
25–44	0.90	4947.1	14.84	14.84	0.0	81626.6	0.0	81626.6
45–64	0.98	4470.7	16.19	16.19	0.0	73766.2	0.0	73766.2
65+	0.82	2812.4	13.49	13.49	0.0	46404.1	0.0	46404.1
$5000–6999								
0– 4	0.33	416.9	5.40	5.40	0.0	6879.7	0.0	6879.7
5–14	0.98	4161.6	16.19	16.19	0.0	68667.1	0.0	68667.1
15–24	1.14	5039.5	18.89	18.89	0.0	83152.1	0.0	83152.1
25–44	0.82	4849.7	13.49	13.49	0.0	80020.0	0.0	80020.0
45–64	0.98	4703.2	16.19	16.19	0.0	77602.6	0.0	77602.6
65+	1.06	2514.6	17.54	17.54	0.0	41491.1	0.0	41491.1

Sample Output from Computer Simulation Program (Continued)

Family Income Age	Visit Rate	Total Visits	Total Expenditure per Capita	Consumer Expenditure per Capita	Federal Expenditure per Capita	Consumer Total Expenditure	Federal Total Expenditure	Total Expenditure
$7000–9999								
0– 4	0.25	483.9	4.05	4.05	0.0	7984.5	0.0	7984.5
5–14	1.39	8111.7	22.93	22.93	0.0	150343.6	0.0	150343.6
15–24	1.55	10469.5	25.63	25.63	0.0	172746.9	0.0	172746.9
25–44	1.14	10345.7	18.89	18.89	0.0	170704.6	0.0	170704.6
45–64	1.14	8207.7	18.89	18.89	0.0	135426.7	0.0	135426.7
65+	1.39	5081.2	22.93	22.93	0.0	83840.2	0.0	83840.2
$10,000–14,999								
0– 4	0.33	1024.2	5.40	5.40	0.0	16899.7	0.0	16899.7
5–14	1.80	18728.9	29.68	29.68	0.0	309026.4	0.0	309026.4
15–24	1.64	17397.4	26.98	26.98	0.0	287057.4	0.0	287057.4
25–44	1.64	23251.1	26.98	26.98	0.0	383642.5	0.0	383642.5
45–64	1.47	16381.7	24.28	24.28	0.0	270297.8	0.0	270297.8
65+	1.06	3656.1	17.54	17.54	0.0	60325.2	0.0	60325.2
$15,000+								
0– 4	0.49	1479.9	8.09	8.09	0.0	24418.8	0.0	24418.8
5–14	2.62	26229.6	43.17	43.17	0.0	432787.8	0.0	432787.8
15–24	2.04	20800.5	33.72	33.72	0.0	343207.7	0.0	343207.7
25–44	1.96	26582.7	32.37	32.37	0.0	438615.0	0.0	438615.0
45–64	2.04	21374.8	33.72	33.72	0.0	352684.1	0.0	352684.1
65+	2.13	5941.1	35.07	35.07	0.0	98028.5	0.0	98028.5
TOTALS		297666.4				4679704.0	231795.6	4911499.0

Epilogue: Summary and Conclusions

The issue of financing dental care is complex and not likely to be resolved to everyone's satisfaction. However, the gap between individual differences might be narrowed if the issues were more sharply focused in a discussion that separated differences in values from differences that are concerned with the costs and the beneficiaries of particular programs. This is what we have attempted to do. Because of lack of data and insufficient knowledge about the effects of some important variables, it has not been possible to be more explicit regarding the costs and the benefits of alternative financing programs.

The approach used in this study on financing dental care was to place dental care in perspective together with other means whereby the community's oral health status might be improved. Practitioners will often make recommendations as to the optimum level of care required to meet the needs within their profession. Economists cannot say whether these optimums ought to be achieved; rather, their role must be to indicate the costs of meeting "optimally" defined levels (or of movements toward meeting them) and compare these to the costs of meeting other needs in health and nonhealth areas. Given the inability to fund all needs in all fields, our ability to allocate dollars to specific needs would be improved if we had better information on the differing costs.

In this spirit we have developed a framework that indicates the choices within the dental sector of some of these alternatives. Specifying the objective of financing programs is the first step in comparing relevant alternatives. Within the broader category of increasing and maintaining oral health status we should ask the question, Which programs have the greater return per additional dollar spent — expenditures on research, dental health education, fluoridation, or dental services?

The data necessary to make comparisons among such broad program categories are not available. One reason for their unavailability is that the objectives and alternatives have not been explicitly defined in dental health. The measurement of how well alternative programs achieve their objectives should be a continual process, since the allocation of funds among programs should respond to changing priorities. The impact of a single program is not constant; at some point, spending funds on alternative programs will result in larger increments per dollar spent toward reaching the policy objective. Therefore, such program comparisons, once developed, should be maintained on a continual basis.

Similar program analyses on a continuous basis should also be made *within* each of the broad program categories affecting oral health. Within the program category of dental services it is possible to achieve a common goal in alternative ways. If, for example, the objective was one of equity — i.e., increasing the use of dental care by certain population groups — then this objective can be achieved either by influencing the demand for dental care or by affecting the supply and availability of such services. Demand and supply policies should thus be viewed as alternatives to one another. (There are, of course, alternative policies within each of the broad categories of supply and demand.)

Unless an objective such as equity is specified and agreed to, it will not be possible to compare seemingly diverse financing programs in dental care. Once an equity objective has been specified, then it is not sufficient merely to suggest that a particular program will achieve that goal; it is important, in evaluating that program, to determine which groups will benefit from it. The actual beneficiaries of government programs are often different from the putative beneficiaries of the program's proposal. And when all programs are classified according to their actual beneficiary groups, the effect on the desired beneficiaries, per dollar spent on each program, may turn out to be quite different from the original expectations.

Unfortunately, when an attempt was made to evaluate one of the largest federal programs in the dental sector, the Health Professions Educational Assistance Act (HPEA), there was insufficient data on both its beneficiaries and its effects. As is the case with many federal programs in medical care, publicly financed programs in dental care "suboptimize"; that is, the goals of such programs are intermediary to the overall objective, which is probably to achieve a redistribution or an increase in care to some population groups. Therefore, what is clearly required for all publicly financed programs in dental care is an information system that would facilitiate comparisons between redistribution programs on the basis of their cost, number and type of beneficiaries, and the amount of care received.

To achieve a better understanding of the effect of alternative financing programs within the dental services sector, and also to judge its performance, three markets and their interrelationships were discussed: the supply and demand for dental care; the derived demands and the supply of dental manpower; and the market for dental and auxiliary training facilities.

In the past, one of the major forces increasing the demand for dental services has been the increase in personal income, which results in greater than proportionate increase in expenditures and use of dental care. There has been some subsidization of the demand for dental care, primarily as a result of Medicaid; however, the magnitude of such governmental support has been less than in other categories of medical care and it has not approached the level requested in many proposals for subsidizing dental care demands.

Off setting these increased demands have been gains in fluoridated water supplies which have undoubtedly decreased dental needs, hence dental demands. On balance, however, there have been increased demands for dental care that when interacting with a relatively nonresponsive supply have caused dental prices to increase almost as rapidly as physician fees.

Forecasts made of the demands and supply of dental services for 1975 suggest that without any further government subsidies of the demands for care, we would expect to observe sufficient increased demands, such that prices should increase by as much as 25 to 32 percent in 1975 over 1970. If, in addition to this continual increase in demand for dental care, there are also large increases in demand as a result of federal financing programs, then the rise in dental care prices, expenditures, and, consequently, the cost of such a program, will be very great. Those people not covered will, in addition to the increased taxes required to fund such a program, face sharply increased prices for dental care. Increased dental prices would decrease demands for care from what they would be otherwise.

Policies that promote fluoridation in the population would decrease demands and thus prevent dental prices from rising as rapidly. The potential gains from fluoridation still appear to be large: more than half the population are without it and only 30 percent of central water systems are fluoridated.

The current limitation to any large financing program for increasing the use of dental services is the responsiveness of the supply of dental care. The importance of supply in any financing program is that it may determine whether or not the financing program will successfully achieve its objective and how much it will cost. If supply doesn't become more responsive to increased demands, then prices will rise sharply and there will be small increases in dental use.

An important determinant of increased supply of dental services over the past twenty years has been the increase in productivity of dentists of about 3 percent per year. The supply of dentists has been increasing by 1.5 percent per year over that same period and expectations are that with federal subsidies to dental schools the number of dentists will increase by 2.0 percent through the current decade. (These figures may overstate the supply of dentists' services since current data indicate that dental hours worked have been decreasing.)

A major policy question with regard to the supply of dental services is: How can the supply of such services be increased even more rapidly so that increased demands for care can be taken care of without large increases in dental prices?

Restrictions prevent auxiliaries from undertaking many dental tasks. Thus the dentist's productivity cannot rise as rapidly as it might. Restrictions on entry into dental schools and on the requirements for becoming a dentist cause the supply of dentists to be smaller than it would be otherwise. Elimination of such restrictions (in full or in part) will increase both the number of dentists and their productivity. Restrictions in dental care inhibit the supply response in each of the several markets. The present supply of dental manpower, and the supply of dental visits, is smaller and the price higher than if there were fewer restrictions.

An analysis of the many restrictions in dental care should be undertaken to determine whether the same quality of dental care (the reason for such restrictions) could be achieved at a lesser cost to society. Although the maintenance and improvement in the quality of dental care is the stated justification for these restrictions, there may also be economic motivations involved in their establishment and continuance. Unless efforts are directed toward measuring the quality of dental care as practiced, it will be difficult to make innovative changes in the "process" of producing well trained manpower. Specifying minimum training periods provides no guarantee that a high quality of care will be performed by the practicing dentist. A more accurate approach for insuring that minimum levels of quality are practiced would be to monitor what is actually practiced. Greater experimentation should then be permitted in the process by which quality dental care is provided. Generally speaking, process restrictions only fulfill the economic motivations that underlie quality barriers. If the motivation was solely one of achieving high quality, then there should be little resistance to removing process restrictions once adequate outcome measures are developed and monitored on a continual basis.

These restrictions, within each of the dental markets, have resulted in a demand for federal and state financing of manpower as a means of increasing the responsiveness of supply to increased demands and needs for dental care.

The role of the government regarding market efficiency in dental care has been to subsidize supply in an attempt to overcome restrictions — which the government itself has sanctioned. It should be noted that the pressure for supply subsidies probably comes from different sources in the dental profession. Existing dentists would probably be opposed to supply subsidies (since it results in an increase in the number of dentists) and would probably favor the loosening of restrictions on use of auxiliaries as the demand for dental care increases — as long as they are under the control of a dentist. The real pressure for supply subsidies most likely comes from the educational institutions.

Large scale federal financing of dental manpower should not be used to lessen the visible effects of restrictions. If the restrictions and their ostensible justifications could be dealt with directly, then federal monies could be used to better advantage in other areas of dental care. The stated basis for federal subsidies to the dental education sector has been the belief of an expected "shortage" of dentists. Estimates of shortage are based on the number of dentists required in some future period to maintain the current dentist to population ratio. In retrospect, estimates of impending shortages have been inaccurate because of incorrect forecasts of population and dental supplies. However since the legislative goals for increasing dentists are tied to specific numbers generated by these forecasts, little flexibility is built into the legislation to revise the funding and goals once more accurate forecasts of population and dental supplies become available.

More important than these technical inadequacies for calculating expected shortages is the conceptual definition of shortages that is used. The ratio technique for estimating shortages fails to incorporate productivity increases, changes in demands for dental services, and does not provide an estimate of the value of decreasing the shortage. By emphasizing numbers of dentists it also precludes from consideration alternatives for achieving the desired social objective — which is, presumably, an increase in dental services to those who cannot afford it.

The equity of providing educational subsidies to the dental sector should also be questioned. Equity in dental care can be analyzed either with respect to the family incomes of students receiving subsidies (in relation to the taxes paid for support of such subsidies), or in a broader context, for achieving greater availability to dental care by different population groups. Subsidies under the Health Professions Educational Assistance Act, 85 percent of which have gone to the dental schools, do not appear to have achieved the equity goal, either broadly or narrowly defined. Under the HPEA students are subsidized in two ways: they receive financial assistance, and their tuition charges are only a small proportion of their costs of education. To date there are no data to indicate that the mix of students in dental schools has changed because of the financial assistance subsidies. Subsidies to dental schools that enable these schools to subsidize their tuition charges benefit all dental students regardless of their family incomes. Tuition that is heavily subsidized also affects the efficiency of the schools' operation and the demand for dental education, as discussed in Chapter 6.

Studies of subsidies to higher education have found that

... sizable numbers of apparently qualified young people (in the upper half of their high school classes) from less affluent families (the bottom two quartiles) do not attend college, while substantial numbers of apparently less qualified young people (in the bottom half of their high schools classes) from more affluent families (the top two quartiles) do attend college. Since financial barriers affect who goes to college and for how long, the current system is nonneutral in its treatment of people.

This nonneutrality results even though tuition averages only about a quarter of the full cost of undergraduate education and large amounts of student financial aid are disbursed. While low tuition reduces the financial barrier for all students, including some to whom full tuition would be no barrier, students from lower-income families may be "able" to attend college only if they obtain additional financial aid to help offset the out-of-pocket costs and, perhaps even more important, the pressure to augment family income (the foregone-earnings costs of college)."[a]

With regard to the equity consideration of increasing dental care to those most needing it — i.e., those persons with low incomes or living in rural areas — subsidies to the dental educational sector do not result in even a significant faction of the funds going for such purposes. As concluded in the analysis of the HPEA, the beneficiaries of the HPEA appear to have been the existing dental schools and the students receiving the subsidies. It would appear that there are more efficient ways to redistribute income and dental care than through

---

[a]W. Lee Hansen, "Equity and the Finance of Higher Education," *Journal of Political Economy.* Part II, May-June, 1972, p. 264.

subsidies to dental education. Subsidies to dental education and the form of those subsidies should be reexamined to determine whether the beneficiaries are those intended, the effects on efficiency are those desired, and the goals of such a program could not be achieved at a lower cost by an alternative program.

Since it does not appear likely that there will be major changes in the structure and organization of dental care delivery in the near future, large price increases will continue, which will raise the financing cost of assisting all those who need dental care, as well as raise the price to those persons not subsidized. These higher prices will undoubtedly cause revisions to be made in the type of financing programs desired; they will either be reduced in scope and/or in the number of beneficiaries. If prices increase greatly with demand type of subsidies then there might also be proposals for extending coverage to other large population groups in order to prevent financial hardships to them. However this would merely exacerbate the problem; it would increase demand and lead to even higher prices.

Similarly, policies might be proposed that would have the effect of separating the subsidized and nonsubsidized markets, e.g., establishing clinics that provide free care. In addition to causing prices to increase more rapidly in the nonsubsidized sector, it would result in two systems for delivering care; an approach that is considered socially undesirable in the rest of the medical care sector. Supply subsidies are likely to be proposed in order to prevent prices from rising so rapidly. However most supply programs are expensive and require years to achieve small increases in output.[b]

It appears therefore that only those subsidy programs that result in the smallest increases in prices and that have the largest degree of public support are most likely to be funded in the next several years. According to a recent survey of public opinion, publicly financed dental programs to low income children have the largest degree of public support.[c]

The probable costs to the government of alternative dental health insurance plans for children vary from a high estimate of five billion dollars to a low estimate of 230 million dollars by 1975, according to whether all children or just low income children are covered. These estimates are presented in the following table.

Limited federal funds and lack of public support suggest that groups outside the low income category are not likely to be covered in the near future. Dental public health programs such as fluoridation and dental health education are not complete substitutes for dental services. However, they do serve to decrease the demand for such services, thus inhibiting the rise in dental prices and enabling

[b]The number of dental graduates in 1965 before the HPEA was 3,200. In 1970 this increased to 3,500. The original goal, which will not be realized, was to reach 6,200 by 1975.

[c]Alice Fusillo and Lois Cohen, "Comparative Analysis of Attitudes Toward Public Dental Care Programs, 1959, 1968," in *ADA Task Force Committee Reports*, pp. 94-96.

the restricted supply of dental services to be used in meeting other demands for dental health care.

Estimates of Alternate Dental Health Insurance Plans for Children for 1970 and 1975

	1970			
	No Plan	Plan 1	Plan 2	Plan 3
Total Visits (000)	$ 305,637.2	319,037.2	339,141.2	534,330.4
Consumer Expend. (000)	3,728,766.0	3,688,506.0	3,628,104.0	2,775,036.0
Federal Expend. (000)	0.0	203,739.6	509,411.0	3,743,789.0
Total Expend. (000)	3,728,766.0	3,892,245.0	4,137,514.0	6,518,821.0

	1975			
	No Plan	Plan 1	Plan 2	Plan 3
Total Visits (000)	285,887.1	297,666.9	314,032.3	517,110.5
Consumer Expend. (000)	4,717,151.0	4,679,711.0	4,627,682.0	3,604,609.5
Federal Expend. (000)	0.0	231,795.8	553,855.2	4,927,561.0
Total Expend. (000)	4,717,151.0	4,911,507.0	5,181,537.0	8,532,162.0

No Plan = Current situation of no federal dental health insurance

Plan 1 = Insurance for all expenses for those in age group 5-14, income class $0-2,999

Plan 2 = Insurance for all expenses for those in age group 5-14, income class $0-2,999 and $3,000-4,999

Plan 3 = Insurance for all expenses for those in age group 0-14, all income classes

"Insurance for all expenses" means those covered face a 0% copay; all those not insured face 100% copay. Assumptions: Elasticity = -0.67; price per visit of care = $12.20 (1970), $16.50 (1975); deductible = 0.

Source: The above estimates were derived using the Dental Health Insurance Computer Simulation Model described in Chapter 6.

Notes

Notes to Chapter 1

1. The description of supply and demand analysis has been necessarily brief. An interested reader can read any one of a number of texts such as R.A. Leftwich, *The Price System and Resource Allocation,* Holt, Rhinehart and Winston, New York: 1970.

It should be kept in mind that the diagrams referred to are "static" in the sense that they show the determination of price and quantity without any other changes occurring in the system. In reality, a great many changes in both demand and supply are occurring so that an equilibrium situation may never actually exist. However, to facilitate the analysis, other factors must be held constant in order to determine the net effect of a change in either demand or supply. In cases where a static analysis would suggest lower dental prices, this should in reality be interpreted to mean lower than they would otherwise have been, since other demand factors are presumably continually working to increase prices.

2. Examples of econometric models in medical care are: M. S. Feldstein, "The Use of an Econometric Model for Health Sector Planning," Discussion Paper No. 14, Harvard Institute for Economic Research, February 1968.

P. J. Feldstein, and S. Kelman, "An Econometric Model of Medical Care Sector," in H. Klarman (Ed.), *Empirical Studies in Health Economics,* Columbia University Press, New York, 1970.

D. E. Yett, L. Drabek, M. D. Intrilligator, and L. J. Kimball, "The Development of a Micro-Simulation Model of Health Manpower Demand and Supply," in *Proceedings and Report of Conference on a Health Manpower Simulation Model,* Department of Health, Education, and Welfare, Washington, D. C., 1970.

Notes to Chapter 2

1. See for example the review articles and accompanying bibliography in this area by N. David Richards, "Utilization of Dental Services," in N. D. Richards and L. K. Cohen, (Eds.), *Social Sciences and Dentistry: A Critical Bibliography,* published by A. Sijthoff, the Hague, Netherlands, 1971.

2. There is a large literature on the effect of fluoridation on tooth decay and costs per child. The following sources are merely indicative of the studies in this area:

David B. Ast, et al., "Time and Cost Factors to Provide Regular, Periodic Dental Care for Children in Fluoridated and Non-Fluoridated Areas: Final Report," *Journal of the American Dental Association,* April 1970. A summary of various studies may be found in *Fluoridation Saves Teeth, Dollars and Dental Manpower,* Division of Dental Health, Department of Health, Education, and Welfare, August 1971; F. J. McClure (Ed.), *Fluoridated Drinking Waters,* U.S. Department of Health, Education and Welfare, 1962; J. R. Blayney, and I.N. Hill, "Fluorine and Dental Caries", *JADA* (special issue), January 1967; I. R. Campbell, *Role of Fluoride in Public Health: The Soundness of Fluoridation in Communal Water Supplies, A Selected Bibliography,* University of Cincinnati, Cincinnati, 1963.

3. Bruce L. Douglas, Donald A. Wallace, Monroe Lerner, and Sylvia Coppersmith, "Impact of Water Fluoridation on Dental Practice and Dental Manpower," *Journal of the American Dental Association,* Vol. 84, February 1972, pp. 355-367.

4. *Water Fluoridation Practices in Major Cities in the United States.* A report prepared for the New York State Department of Health by the New York University College of Engineering. See p. 54, Table 15. For the 18 cities studied, the annual operating costs for fluoridation varied from $.018 per capita to $.12 per capita.

Other means of achieving the benefits of fluoridation are available to the consumer, such as taking fluoride pills, but at a higher cost than $0.10 per year per person.

5. It has been argued that fluoridation only postpones rather than eliminates expenditures on dental care by keeping people in the market for dental care for a much longer period, and that fluoridation may even increase dental expenditures in the long run, by preserving the teeth so that expensive peridontal treatment, bridges, and partial dentures will be needed before full dentures are finally fitted in any case. (See "The Need and the Demand for Dental Care," Walter T. Pelton, and Ruth D. Bothwell, Public Health Analyst, Manpower and Education Branch, Division of Dental Public Health and Resources, U.S. Public Health Service, in *Proceedings of the Workshop on Future Requirements on Dental Manpower and the Training and Utilization of Auxiliary Personnel,* University of Michigan, Ann Arbor, 1962.)

Assuming this were true, such increased long-term expenditures on dental care would be the result, not of fluoridation itself, but rather of increased income. If income were too low to allow for increased dental expenditures, fluoridation would postpone loss of teeth without entailing further dental expenditures.

6. The data for this analysis was based on data from the American Dental Association's *Survey of Dental Practice.* The method of estimation was two stage least squares. A more complete description of this model and its applications is presented in Chapter 5, "An Econometric Model of the Dental Sector." The statistical results of the demand equation are as follows:

	Constant Term	Income	Price	R^2	N
	1302.40	1.221*	−258.97*	.86	35
		(.086)**	(27.39)**		
(Logarithms)	−1.51	1.713*	−1.431*	.86	35

*Significant at .005 level
**Standard error

Sources:

Mean Annual Patient Visits per Dentist: American Dental Association, *The Survey of Dental Practice,* 1956, 1959, 1962, 1965, 1968.

Mean Gross Income of Dentists: *Ibid.* ("Price per Visit" calculated as "Mean Gross Income of Dentists" ÷ "Mean Annual Patient Visits per Dentist". "Mean Gross Income of Dentists" calculated as "Mean Net Income of all Dentists" ÷ "Mean Net Income as Percent of Mean Gross Income of Independent Dentists".)

Total Active Dentist: ADA, *Distribution of Dentists in the United States by State, Region, District and County,* 1956, 1959, 1962, 1966, 1969 (not published in 1967-1968; thus 1967 figures are weighted averages of 1965 and 1968 figures).

Civilian Population: U.S. Bureau of the Census, *Current Population Reports,* Series P-25, Nos. 304, 348, and 414. ("Dental Visits per 1000 Population" calculated as "Total Active Dentists" ÷ "1000 Civilian Population" X "Mean Annual Patient Visits per Dentist.")

Per Capita Income: U.S. Bureau of the Census, *Statistical Abstract of the United States* (various editions).

7. An earlier independent study based on different national data, which was derived from the 1958 HIF survey, produced roughly the same results. It was concluded that "for a 10 percent increase in income, expenditures on dental care will rise by approximately 12 percent." American Medical Association, *Report of the Commission on the Cost of Medical Care.* Vol. 1, General Report, Paul J. Feldstein, "Demand for Medical Care," p. 69.

8. The empirical estimates of the effect of income on the demand for dental care have, because of lack of data, excluded other factors believed to have an effect on demand. Since these excluded variables may change the income effect if they were to be included, some estimates of this possible change would be desirable. There is some evidence available to suggest that while the inclusion of these other variables will decrease the effect of income, that the permanent income hypothesis for dental care is supported and that the income elasticity is approximately "one." Based on national data collected in 1964 by the National Opinion Research Center, Andersen and Benham found that the income elasticity was 1.24 when other variables were not included and .99 when they were. (The regression coefficients were .009 and .008 respectively.) Ronald Andersen and Lee Benham, "Factors Affecting the Relationship Between Family Income and Medical Care Consumption," in H. Klarman (Ed.), *Empirical Studies in Health Economics,* The Johns Hopkins Press, Baltimore, Maryland, 1970.

9. In a recently published study, C. Upton and W. Silverman ("The Demand for Dental Services," *The Journal of Human Resources,* Spring 1971) also derived estimates of the income elasticity of demand for dental services. An

interesting aspect of their study was their attempt to estimate the income elasticity of demand for different types of dental services. They find that there are substantial differences in the income effect between types of services. For example those dental services that are more highly related to increased income (i.e., income elasticity greater than one) are restorations-deciduous teeth, inlays, crowns, jackets, bridges, and dentures.

10. In the Upton-Silverman article, op. cit., estimates were also made of the effect of fluoridation on the demands for different types of dental treatment and the present value of savings on dental expenditures for selected services. Their findings indicate that decreases in restorations, bridges, and dentures have the highest return, with extractions and prophylactic treatments next, when water supplies are fluoridated.

11. There have however been several studies which have attempted to assess the impact of various public programs. See for example:

A. Jong, and G. Leske, "Utilization and Cost of Dental Services for Pre-School Children in Boston's Head Start Program," *Journal of Public Health Dentistry,* Spring 1968.

H. Zipporah, and E. Leatherwood, "A Dental Program for Head Start Children in New York City; A Retrospective Study of Utilization and Costs," *Medical Care,* July-August 1969.

Blanche E. Ross, "A comparative Study of Four Dental Payments Mechanisms in a Head Start Program," *American Journal of Public Health,* Vol. 61, No. 11, November 1971, pp. 2176-2187.

I. Brightman, and N. Allaway, "Evaluation of Medical and Dental Care Under the Medical Assistance Program," *American Journal of Public Health,* December 1969.

R. M. O'Shea, J. F. Rosner, G. D. Bissell, and D. W. Johnston, "The Impact of Medicaid on Dental Practice: Some Evidence from Erie County, New York," *New York Dental Journal,* November 1969.

12. For an excellent discussion of "moral hazard" with respect to insurance for medical care, see the article by Mark Pauly, "The Economics of Moral Hazard: Comment," *American Economic Review,* June 1968.

13. For a discussion of dentists' attitudes in this area, see Robert C. Jones, "Dentist's View on Reimbursement Arrangements Under Prepayment and Insurance Plans," *Journal of the American Dental Association,* Vol. 84, No. 1, January 1972, pp. 125-129.

14. This aspect is discussed more fully in the article by M. V. Pauly, op. cit.

15. Still another approach recently reported on is to provide an incentive to the enrollee in the form of reduced coinsurance if he receives annual dental attention. Washington Dental Service reports lower treatment cost per patient in their third and fourth years compared to those in their first two years. "Dental Insurance Is Different," *Journal of the American Dental Association,* October 1971, p. 754.

16. As an example of one approach to develop a forecasting model for dental premiums, given the characteristics of the enrolled group, see B. V. Dean, U. N. Bhat, A. J. Singh, and C. Das, *Prepaid Dental Plan: Final Report,* Technical Memorandum No. 141, Operations Research Department, School of Management, Case Western Reserve University, February 1969.

Notes to Chapter 3

1. Arlene S. Holen, "Effects of Professional Licensing Arrangements on Interstate Labor Mobility and Resource Allocation," *Journal of Political Economy,* October 1965; L. Benham, A. Maurizi, and M. Reder, "Migration, Location and Remuneration of Medical Personnel: Physicians and Dentists," *Review of Economics and Statistics,* August 1968.

2. L. Benham, A. Maurizi, and M. Reder, op. cit., p. 346.

3. These observations are also made in the article by A. Holen, op. cit., p. 497.

4. In discussions of dental care, reference is made to both population-dentist and dentist-population ratios. For purposes of consistency, population-dentist ratios are used throughout this paper. However for comparative purposes in those instances when dentist-population ratios are used elsewhere, the following two series are presented:

Population:Dentist Ratio	Dentists:Population Ratio (per thousand population)
2174:1	.46
2084:1	.48
2000:1	.50
1923:1	.52
1852:1	.54
1786:1	.56
1275:1	.58

5. These are dentists as listed in Immigration and Naturalization Service Reports as "Immigrants by occupation . . . dentists." U.S. Department of Justice, Immigration and Naturalization Service, *Annual Reports.*

6. In W. Young, and D. Striffler, *The Dentist, His Practice and His Community,* second ed., W. B. Saunders Co., Philadelphia, 1969, p. 273, the authors report, based on a study, that there were an additional 4,000 dentists in 1965 who had "informally limited" their practice. Thus the actual number of specialists would be greater than the data indicate.

7. *Survey of Dental Practice,* op. cit., 1968.

8. According to data from various issues of the ADA's *Survey of Dental Practice,* the average hours worked per year by the dentist was:

1970	1949.0	1958	2090.4
1967	2023.8	1955	2039.0
1964	2039.0	1952	2013.5
1961	2038.3		

9. J. Jeffers has cautioned too great a reliance on productivity estimates based on such aggregate data. "If . . . case mix remains constant over time, then increased number of patient visits accompanying greater use of dental auxiliaries, with hours worked remaining constant, reflect increased dental productivity. This would not be the case, however, if quality of output declined or if the character of dental services rendered per visit changes over time . . .If auxiliaries are hired to produce additional services such as scaling, teeth cleaning, and the teaching of fundamentals of oral hygiene, then increased patient visits per dentist do not reflect increased dental productivity, but rather reflects increased diversification of dental output and merely an expansion of output that is attributable to the performing of additional services by dental auxiliaries."

Current data, unfortunately, do not permit us to examine the case mix of different combinations of dentists and auxiliaries.

10. J. Weiss, *The Changing Job Structure of Health Manpower,* unpublished Doctoral Dissertation, Harvard University, Cambridge, Mass., 1966.

11. A. Maurizi, *Economic Essays on the Dental Profession,* op. cit., pp. 66-67.

12. *Survey of Dentistry,* op. cit., p. 478.

13. A. Maurizi, op. cit., pp. 68-69.

14. Maurizi (op. cit.) estimated a production function for nonsalaried dentists and found that there are increasing returns to dental practice. The sum of the coefficients of the three factor inputs — annual hours worked by the dentist, the number of assistants, and the number of chairs in the office — is approximately 1.50 (p. 59). The economic interpretation of this finding is that the dentist will realize a more than proportionate return from his increased use of these factor inputs.

15. For a discussion of the effect of marginal revenue on work effort as applied to physicians in group practice, see Joseph Newhouse, "The Economics of Group Practice," The Rand Corporation, 1971 (memeo).

16. See Donald Yett, "An Evaluation of Methods of Estimating Physician's Expenses Relative to Output," *Inquiry,* March 1967; and Richard Bailey, "Economies of Scale in Medical Practice," in H. Klarman (Ed.), *Empirical Studies in Health Economics,* The Johns Hopkins Press, Baltimore, Md., 1970.

17. ADA *Survey of Dental Practice,* 1968, p. 35.

18. *Royal Commission on Health Services,* Vol. 2, 1964, p. 573. However, David A. Soricelli, "Practical Experience in Peer Review Controlling Quality in

the Delivery of Dental Care," *American Journal of Public Health,* October 1971, describes a dental team that consists of one dentist, one hygienist, four technotherapists, two dental assistants, and one clerk. See page 2053.

19. The Manpower Committee of the Task Force on National Health Programs of the American Dental Association has also made forecasts of dental visit capacity for 1970 and 1975 (American Dental Association, Task Force on National Health Programs, "The Requirements for Dental and Dental Auxiliary Manpower," *Dentistry in National Health Programs: Reports of the Special Committees,* Chicago, 1971). These are based on an assumption of a 3.5 percent annual increase in dentist productivity, plus an additional 10 percent increase in productivity between 1970 and 1980. At their assumed productivity levels, the Manpower Committee's visit capability forecasts are 371,400,000 in 1970 (3,745 per dentist) and 437,300,000 in 1975 (4,075 per dentist).

Additionally, the Manpower Committee has made alternative forecasts based on greater use by dentists of expanded function auxiliaries, assuming necessary legal changes. The assumptions here are that EFA's would be used primarily by new dental graduates; that half the dentists using EFA's would increase their productivity by 80 percent by using three auxiliaries; and that the other half of the dentists would increase their productivity by 130 percent using four auxiliaries. On this basis, a 1975 visit capability of 449,111,000 total visits (4,185 per dentist) is forecast.

20. See, for example, the review and bibliography in this area by Alice E. Fusillo and A. Stafford Metz, "Social Science Research on the Dental Student," in N. D. Richards and L. K. Cohen, Editors, *Social Sciences and Dentistry: A Critical Bibliography,* published by A. Sijthoff, The Hague, Netherlands, 1971.

Notes to Appendix 3A

1. These calculations are based upon the regression equations developed by Alex R. Maurizi in "Migration of Dentists," *Economic Essays on the Dental Profession,* University of Iowa, 1969. See especially Regression Table II-2, p. 43.

2. *Report of the Committee on Labor and Public Welfare, United States Senate,* on S. 934, July 12, 1971. U.S. Government Printing Office, Washington, D.C., 1971, p. 8.

3. *Hearings Before the Subcommittee on Public Health and Environment of the Committee on Interstate and Foreign Commerce, House of Representatives,* 92nd Congress, 1st Session, on H.R. 703, 4171, 4155, 5614, 5767, 7765, 4145, 4156, 5618, 7707, 7736, April 2, 3, 20, 21, 22, 27, 28, 29, 1971. Statement of Dr. James Bowden, Dean, University of North Carolina School of Dentistry, in behalf of the American Dental Association and American Association of Dental Schools; accompanied by Dr. Richard K. Mosbaugh, Chairman, Council on Legislation, ADA, and Hal M. Christensen, Director, Washington Office, ADA, U.S. Government Printing Office, Washington, D.C., 1971, p. 717.

4. *Report of the Committee on Labor and Public Welfare,* op. cit.

5. Percentage of dentists practicing in same state in which they graduated from dental school, by ADA region, 1964 and 1970.

Region	1964	1970
New England	52.3%	51.2%
Middle East	51.7	49.4
Southeast	43.8	46.2
Southwest	77.0	78.1
Central	54.0	52.3
Northwest	35.7	33.3
Far West	76.4	77.3
United States	54.4	53.6

Source: 1964, Bureau of Economic Research and Statistics, "Inventory of Dentists — 1964," *Journal of the American Dental Association,* Vol. 70, May 1965, pp. 1261-1269. 1970, unpublished data from the Bureau of Economic Research and Statistics, American Dental Association.

Notes to Chapter 4

1. Various issues of *The Survey of Dental Practice,* op. cit., and the *Statistical Abstract of the United States.*

2. It has been estimated that the number of dental assistants trained on the job are approximately 12,000 per year. R. Castaldi, "Dental Auxiliaries: Dentistry's Dilemma," *Journal of the American Dental Association,* May 1972, p. 1080.

"Requirements for Approval of a Certifying Board for Dental Assistants" was accepted by the American Dental Association in 1960. Dental assistants who completed a special 104-hour educational program before 1967 were eligible for examination until 1969. Since 1969, M.A. candidates for examination by the Certifying Board must have completed an accredited educational pro- gram . . . [such] programs [should] be at least one academic year in length and be conducted in an accredited post-high school educational institution. "Report of the Inter-Agency Committee on Dental Auxiliaries," *JADA,* May 1972, p. 1029.

3. As long as there is excess demand for a dental education presumably a school could charge full costs (and more) and still survive. However it would probably be difficult for such a school to be accredited. Dr. Mann (*Survey of Dentistry*) states, "The greatest influence of the Gies report [William J. Gies' 1926 report on dental education] lies in the demise of the proprietary schools, although for this the Dental Educational Council of America perhaps deserves part of the credit . . ." pp. 243-244). "Early in the decade beginning in 1901, disgust with the quality of many of the dental schools, and opposition to increase in their number, became very general, and their multiplication was abruptly halted" (statement by W. J. Gies on p. 244 of Dr. Mann's article).

4. *The Annual Report on Dental Auxiliary Education 1970/71,* published by the American Dental Association, provides data by school on enrollments, admission requirements, length of course, school capacity, percent of capacity filled, etc., for all schools offering training in dental assisting, dental hygiene, and dental laboratory technology. The percentage of first-year places filled were 78 percent for dental hygiene, 80 percent for laboratory technicians, and 86 percent for dental assisting. Within each of these educational areas, those schools with lower admission requirements and/or shorter training time had a higher percentage of their capacity filled.

5. Table 5, pp. 10-13, *Manpower Supply and Educational Statistics,* PHS publications No. 263, section 20 (as of March 1971).

6. William R. Mann, "Dental Education," in Byron S. Hollinshead *Survey of Dentistry,* American Council on Education, Washington, D.C., 1961, p. 294.

7. It is interesting to note that although educational cost per student is higher in public dental schools, the costs to *students* of attending dental schools (including tuition, fees, books, etc.) are higher in private dental schools than for those attending public dental schools. *The Health Professions Educational Assistance Program: Report to the President and Congress,* U.S. Department of Health, Education, and Welfare, Washington, D.C., September 1970, p. 92.

8. Under the amendments to the HPEA program passed in November 1971, Public Law 92-157, evaluations are now to be made of the use of the monies granted to schools under the program. Specifically, studies of the cost of construction of health facilities and of average cost per year of educating health professions students are to be undertaken. The National Academy of Sciences is to conduct these studies. In addition, the National Academy of Sciences is to make recommendations as to how the federal government can most equitably make capitation grants to schools on the basis of these costs. The 1971 amendments to the HPEA include incentives to the schools to reduce training times: for example, a four-year school can receive a maximum of $11,500 per graduated student, over a four-year period, while a school that graduates a student in three years will receive $13,500 per student over the three-year period. It will be interesting to observe how many schools take advantage of this financial inducement. U.S. Congress, Senate, *Conference Report to Accompany H.R. 8629,* Report No. 92-398, October 19, 1971, p. 34.

9. U.S. Congress, House of Representatives, *Hearings Before the Committee on Interstate and Foreign Commerce on H.R. 4999, H.R. 8774 and H.R. 8833,* Summary Statement of the American Dental Association, p. 178, January 23, 24, 25, 26, and 30, 1962, U.S. Government Printing Office, Washington, D.C., 1962.

10. U.S. Congress, Senate, *Hearings before the Subcommittee on Health of the Committee on Labor and Public Welfare, on S. 911 and H.R. 12,* August 22, 23, 26, 1963, Statement of Boisfeuillet Jones, Special Assistant for Health and Medical Affairs, U.S. Department of Health, Education, and Welfare, accom-

panied by Dr. Luther Terry, Surgeon General, U.S. Public Health Service, p. 69, U.S. Government Printing Office, Washington, D.C., 1963.

These loan and scholarship grants have increased over time. Under the amendments to HPEA passed in Public Law 92-157 (November 1971), loan grants and scholarship grants are both given to schools in the amount of $3,000 times one-tenth the number of full-time students enrolled, or $3,000 times the number of full-time students enrolled who are from low-income backgrounds (see below). U.S. Congress, Senate, *Conference Report to Accompany H.R. 8629,* Report No. 92-398, October 19, 1971, p. 57. The maximum yearly value of the loan or scholarship which may be received by a student is now $3,500 (with certain exceptions as noted below). *Conference Report,* ibid., pp. 22, 24.

11. Statement of Honorable Abraham Ribicoff, Secretary, accompanied by Wilbur J. Cohen, Assistant Secretary, Boisfeuillet Jones, Special Assistant to the Secretary, Health and Medical Affairs, and Dr. Luther L. Terry, Surgeon General, Public Health Service, Department of Health, Education, and Welfare, in *Hearings . . . on H.R. 4999, H.R. 8774, and H.R. 8833,* op. cit., p. 21.

12. Under Public Law 92-157, specific policies have been incorporated into the HPEA program with the intention of increasing the percentage of health professions students coming from lower socioeconomic backgrounds. In particular, federal grants to schools, scholarship and loan funds, which were originally based on school enrollment only, are now to be calculated on the basis of "$3,000 times the number of full-time students enrolled who are from low income backgrounds or $3,000 times one-tenth of the number of full-time students enrolled, whichever is higher." (It would be interesting to determine the number of schools that select this latter option for receiving federal funds. If many dental schools were to base their calculations on total enrollment rather than on the number of students from low income backgrounds, then the basis for providing such student financial support would have been subverted.) Additionally, whereas the maximum yearly loan or scholarship has been set at $3,500, the maximum may be raised to $5,000 for students who are from lower socioeconomic backgrounds or if they are residents of physician shortage areas. (It would appear that the relevant criteria for who receives the larger scholarship should not be the background of the student but where the student practices once he graduates. In any case, data should be collected to determine whether low income students in fact return to low income areas to practice.) Loan forgiveness provisions have been instituted for health professions students who are "from a low income or disadvantaged family." Finally, special grants have been made available to "assist schools of medicine, osteopathy, dentistry, veterinary medicine, optometry, pharmacy, and podiatry in meeting the costs of special projects to . . . establish and operate projects designed to increase admissions to and enrollment in such schools of qualified individuals from minority or low income groups." See *Conference Report to Accompany H.R. 8629,* op. cit., pp. 16, 22, 27, 57.

13. U.S. Congress, Senate, *Report of the Committee on Labor and Public Welfare on S. 934,* July 12, 1971, U.S. Government Printing Office, Washington, D.C., 1971, p. 8.

14. Ibid., p. 23.

15. Supplementary statement of the American Dental Association in *Hearings,* January 23, 1962, op. cit., p. 182.

16. U.S. Congress, Senate, *Report of the Committee on Labor and Public Welfare on S. 934,* July 12, 1971. U.S. Government Printing Office, Washington, D.C., 1971, p. 10. It is interesting to note that the amended HPEA of 1971 (Public Law 92-157) makes special provision for grants designed specifically to assist schools which are in financial distress. *Conference Report to Accompany H.R. 8629,* op. cit., p. 17.

17. Supplementary statement of the American Dental Association, in *Hearings,* January 23, 1962, op. cit., p. 182.

18. Attempts have been made in the amendments to the HPEA to tie these grants to required enrollment increases. For example, in order to receive a grant "to improve the quality" of the school, such school must accompany its application with "reasonable assurances . . . that for the first school year in which such grant is first made and/or each school year thereafter during which such a grant is made the first-year enrollment of full-time students in such school will exceed the number of such students enrolled in the school year beginning during the fiscal year ending June 30, 1971 (i) by 10 per centum of each such number if such number was not more than 100, or (ii) by 5 per centum of such number, or 10 students, whichever is greater, if such number was more than 100." It is also possible for a school to receive up to an additional $150,000 per class per year by exceeding the above requirements, in which case it will receive $1,000 per student for each student above the minimum. New schools, in order to receive "start up assistance," must have at least 24 students in their initial first-year classes. Public Law 92-157, 92nd Congress, H.R. 8629, November 18, 1971, pp. 8, 10, 13. These provisions will supposedly force schools to increase enrollments, and should serve as an inducement to schools to expand their operations and thus operate closer to the "minimum cost" point on their "average cost of education per student" curve.

However, schools with a first-year student enrollment of less than 51 may receive an additional grant of $50,000 per year (Public Law 92-157, op. cit., p. 8). While this provision is an obvious benefit to new schools just beginning their operations, it also serves as an inducement to these schools and for existing small schools *not* to expand to a point "farther out" on the average cost curve. Thus, this provision seems to work in opposition to the two enrollment tied clauses described above.

It should be interesting to observe whether schools take advantage of these funds, and whether total student enrollment increases by at least 10 percent a year.

19. *Health Manpower Source Book,* op. cit., p. 38.

20. Ibid.

21. Statement of Raymond J. Nagle, Dean, College of Dentistry, New York University, and Chairman, American Dental Association Council on Dental Education (in *Hearings* of January 23, 1962, op. cit., p. 172).

The 1972 amended program, however, provides for increases in the Federal share. Specifically, "the Federal share shall not exceed 80 percent on projects for new schools, or for new facilities for existing schools providing a major expansion of training capacity, and that the Federal share shall not exceed 70 percent for any other project, except in the cases of unusual circumstances, not to exceed 80 percent and on major remodeling to meet an increase in student enrollment." *Conference Report to Accompany H.R. 8629,* op. cit., p. 44.

22. *Health Manpower Source Book,* op. cit., p. 7 (1970 figures), p. 8 (1975 estimates).

In 1961-1962 total enrollment was 13,513 from 47 schools. In 1969-1970 total enrollment was 16,008 from 53 schools. Of the 2,495 additional enrollment, 742 came from the six new schools with the remainder (1,753) from the existing schools. (During the last several years (1970 and 1971) two existing schools closed.)

23. The "expert groups" which Dr. Nagle said had scrutinized dentistry and its professional manpower, and the reports of these groups, are as follows:

1. "Medical School Inquiry" staff report to the Committee on Interstate and Foreign Commerce, House of Representatives, 85th Congress, 1st session (committee print).

2. U.S. Department of Health, Education, and Welfare, Office of the Secretary, "The Advancement of Medical Research and Education through the Department of Health, Education, and Welfare: Final Report of the Secretary's Consultants on Medical Research and Education, 1958" (the Bayne-Jones report).

3. U.S. Department of Health, Education, and Welfare, Public Health Service, "Physicians for a Growing America: Report of the Surgeon General's Consultant Group on Medical Education, 1959" (the Bane report).

4. Subcommittee on Departments of Labor, Health, Education, and Welfare of the Committee of Appropriations; U.S. Senate (86th Congress, 2nd Session), "Federal Support of Medical Research: Report of the Committee of Consultants on Medical Research, 1960."

5. American Council on Education, Commission on the Survey of Dentistry in the United States, "The Survey of Dentistry, 1961."

24. The basis for the different productivity estimates, which is described more completely in the sections on productivity and supply, are as follows: the estimate of one percent annual increase in productivity caused by technical change is a result of separate studies by A. Maurizi, op. cit., and B. Hollingshead,

op. cit. The annual productivity increase of 3 percent is approximately that for all factors affecting dental productivity based on our calculations of the increase in visits per dentist for the period 1950-1970. J. Weiss, in his study which was based on total real expenditures for dental care over the period 1950-1963, also derived a 3 percent annual increase in dental productivity.

25. An analysis of loan forgiveness provisions with respect to physicians found that, "It is significant that only one program has had outstanding success over its 25-year history, while the majority of states are fortunate if 60 percent of the borrowing physicians follow through by practicing in the rural areas of their states. In all of these programs, one-third of the physicians chose to buy out of their obligation to practice in a small community." (Henry R. Mason, "Effectiveness of Student Aid Programs Tied to a Service Commitment," *Journal of Medical Education,* July, 1971, p. 576.)

Nevertheless, Public Law 92-157 includes a loan forgiveness provision for health professions students. Under this provision a graduate may be forgiven up to 85 percent of his loan by practicing up to three years in a personnel-shortage area. Also, the maximum loan or scholarship which a student agreeing to practice in a shortage area may receive is set at $5,000 per year, as opposed to the "normal" ceiling of $3,500 per year. Further, special grants are available to schools in "meeting the costs of special projects to establish and operate projects designed to identify and increase admissions to and enrollment in schools . . . of, individuals whose background and interests make it reasonable to assume that they will engage in the practice of their health profession in rural or other areas having a severe shortage of personnel." *Conference Report to Accompany H.R. 8629,* op. cit., p. 16.

Notes to Appendix 4A

1. Under Public Law 92-157, the National Academy of Sciences, which is to study the use of HPEA monies are to "develop methodologies for ascertaining the national average annual per student educational costs" and "indicate the extent of the variation among schools within the respective disciplines in their annual per student educational costs and the key factors affecting this variation." Furthermore, the study groups are also to "describe national uniform standards for determining annual per student educational costs for each health professional school in future years." *Conference Report to accompany H.R. 8629,* op. cit., p. 35. Hopefully, this will result in the development of an accurate average cost curve for dental schools.

Notes to Chapter 5

1. The primary source for much of the data was American Dental Association publications. Data on price of dental visits, number of patient visits,

hours worked by dentists, dentist incomes, and auxiliary personnel came from the *Surveys of Dental Practice* published in 1956, 1959, 1962, 1965, and 1968. The observations used in the statistical analyses consisted of the seven regions (as defined by the ADA) of the United States for each of those years. There were thus seven observations from each of five years, giving a total of thirty-five observations. Data on the stock of dentists came from *The Distribution of Dentists in the United States by state, region, district, and county,* issues for the above years (or straight line interpolation for years when *The Distribution of Dentists* was not published). Demographic data on population, age distribution, mortality rates, and income came from standard Bureau of the Census sources such as *The Statistical Abstract of the United States* and *Current Population Reports.* Data on dental school spaces, enrollments, dropouts, and graduates came from various Department of Health, Education, and Welfare Public Health Service publications. Finally, data on school construction costs were derived from the actual average cost incurred by construction projects financed by the Health Professions Education Act.

2. This function has been estimated by Alex R. Maurizi ("Production Function for the Dental Service Industry," *Economic Essays on the Dental Profession,* The University of Iowa, Iowa City, Iowa, 1967) using dental practice survey data for 1961. Apparently Maurizi was allowed by the ADA to examine the actual survey replies for that year, thus enabling him to make a cross section estimation of a production function.

Maurizi also attempted an analysis of the determinants of the number of annual hours worked per dentist (HRD). His equation, for dentists of all ages (equations have also been estimated by age groups), is:

$$HRD = 2413.7 + 26.8\,AWA + 65.5\,AUX - 30.8\,WR - 6.4\,PRO - 6.5\,AGE$$
$$R^2 = .12$$

where AWA = average wait in days by a patient to get an appointment; AUX = number of full-time auxiliaries employed per dentist; $WR = \dfrac{\text{annual net income}}{\text{annual hours}}$; PRO = fee for prophylaxis; AGE = age of dentist.

In the course of constructing the model, we also estimated an "hours per dentist" equation, regressing it simultaneously with the supply and demand equations. This equation was:

$$HRD = 2134.98 - 10.86\,WR$$
$$R^2 = .33$$

Our equation used the "average net wage per hour worked" as the measure of both price and income, whereas Maurizi used a separate price variable (both results are statistically significant).

Two points should be noted in comparing the equations. First, both show HRD to vary inversely with the "average net wage per hour worked." Second, the point elasticity of WR for Maurizi's equation, calculated at the 1961 means of HRD and WR (2038.3 and $7.63) is $-.12$; while for our equation (which used cross section observations over time) it is $-.04$ (means = 2045.5 and $8.24).

The interpretation of these elasticities is that the supply of dental hours is unresponsive to higher prices for dental care. (Higher prices would actually reduce the number of dental hours worked.) Therefore, with increased prices for dental care and a given number of dentists, increased output would have to come from increasing the dentist's productivity.

3. Subsequent to the estimation and application of the above model, data from the 1970 *Survey of Dental Practice* was published in the *JADA*. When the parameters were reestimated, incorporating the additional observations, the results were not significantly different. A minor difference was in the price elasticity of supply; it was slightly lower (from .29 to .21) with the additional observations. When forecasts were made for 1975 using the new reduced forms, the price of a visit was slightly higher and utilization slightly lower.

Because the parameters and results derived using the new data do not differ substantially from the original estimates and because of the illustrative nature of the forecasts, policy, and sensitivity analyses which were conducted, it was decided to present the simulations in terms of the originally estimated model.

4. The estimate of net income being 53 percent of gross income is from the ADA's *Survey of Dental Practice,* 1967, p. 11.

5. For an example of a more detailed application of the ratio technique, see Bureau of Economic Research and Statistics, "Number of Dental Graduates Required Annually to 1985," *Journal of the American Dental Association,* Vol. 71, September 1969, pp. 694-698. The basis of this application was a goal of maintaining the 1963 dentist-population ratio (1:1,988) in 1985.

In this article, four Bureau of the Census population projections (series A, B, C, and D) for 1985 were used and the authors calculated the total active dentists which would be necessary under each population assumption to maintain the 1963 dentist-population ratio in 1985. Next, using mortality rates of white males in 1962 and defining a "professionally active dentist" as "a dentist younger than 68 years of age," they computed how many of the current year stock of dentists would remain alive and in active practice in each year through 1985. Finally, assuming that the annual increase in dental graduates would be uniform from year to year, the number of dental graduates required in each year 1969-1985 to bring the supply of dentists up to the point such that the dentist-population ratio was 1:1,988 in 1975, 1980 and 1985 was calculated for each population projection. A formula was presented for calculating the required annual increase in dental school graduates and the required yearly graduates in order to have the dentist-population ratio reach any particular level by 1985.

6. The forecast of the stock of active practicing dentists in 1975 produced by the econometric model simulation may be compared with estimates found in other sources. The Division of Manpower Intelligence, Bureau of Health Manpower Education, in *Projections of Manpower Resources in Selected Health Professions, 1970-1980* (Report No. 72-58, February 1972), forecast a stock of 112,920 practicing dentists in 1975. This estimate does not include the net additions (graduates minus deaths) in 1975, while the model includes these. Thus the model forecast for 1975 (110,980 active practicing dentists) should be compared to the DMI forecast for 1976 (115,530).

The Division of Manpower Intelligence used the following assumptions in making their forecasts: (1) Existing HPEA legislation would be extended to fiscal year 1977 in its 1971 form and at approximately its 1971 levels of support. (The model also used roughly this same assumption.) (2) The figures used for graduates for 1972, 1973, 1974 were the number reported by schools on their fiscal year 1971 institutional grant applications as being fourth year students, updated from information supplied by schools to the Bureau of Health Manpower Education on curriculum shortening. Graduates for 1975 were computed from first-year students four years earlier, using a dropout rate of 5 percent, plus an additional output of 100 graduates due to curriculum shortening. The model employed similar methodology, but used a 10 percent dropout rate and made no provisions for curriculum shortening. (3) Deaths were calculated using an overall annual death rate of .017, which was derived by applying the death rates by age groups for white males in 1967 to the number of dentists in each age group as of 1968. This death rate (.017) was applied to the total number of dentists (active and inactive) in each year. The model used a coefficient of .020 in the number of active practicing dentists in each year to determine deaths and retirements. (4) The net addition to the total number of dentists in each year was calculated as dental graduates minus deaths for that year. This figure was added to the total number of dentists in the year to obtain the total number of dentists in the following year. Finally, the number of active practicing dentists for that (following) year was obtained by taking 88 percent of the total stock of dentists. This 88 percent figure therefore includes an implicit estimate of the amount of yearly retirees from active practice. The model simulations worked only in terms of active dentists, and considered retirements with deaths, as mentioned above.

Another set of estimates of the supply of dentists is found in *Health Manpower Source Book: Section 20, Manpower Supply and Educational Statistics* (PHS Publication No. 263, updated to March 3, 1971), which was prepared by the Manpower Studies Branch, Division of Dental Health. They estimate 111,400 active practicing dentists in 1975. These estimates are comparable to the same years used in the econometric model forecasts. The Division of Dental Health estimates assumed that construction funds for dental schools would be $23,000,000 annually under the HPEA. These federal construction subsidies were assumed to be at the rate of $28,000,000 per year in the econometric model.

7. In 1962, the average salary of the 77,500 employed hygienists, technicians and assistants was $3,290. In 1965, the 95,400 auxiliaries averaged $3,691 and in 1967, the 111,200 auxiliaries received an average salary of $4,355. (Source: *Survey of Dental Practice*, 1962, 1965, and 1968. The figure for each year is an overall average of the average salaries of hygienists, technicians, and assistants in each year, weighted by the number of each type of auxiliary in each year.) If it is assumed that salaries increased by an additional 15 percent between 1968 and 1970 then the mean wage would be $5,000 per year.

8. These calculations are: 1.4305 X 1.0193 = 1.4581 auxiliaries per dentist. (1.4581 −1.4305)(109,537), 109,537 is the number of dentists without the HPEA program in 1975. This equals 3,023 auxiliaries. Assuming the annual wage for an auxiliary in 1975 is approximately $7,000, then $7,000 x 3,023 = $21,161,610.

Notes to Chapter 6

1. For a more complete discussion of externalities and public goods, see, for example, James M. Buchanan, *The Demand and Supply of Public Goods,* Rand McNally and Company, Chicago, 1968; Richard A. Musgrave, *The Theory of Public Finance,* McGraw Hill Book Company, New York, 1959; Paul A. Samuelson, "The Pure Theory of Public Expenditure," *Review of Economics and Statistics,* November 1954.

2. For an excellent discussion of the various criteria used in cost-benefit analyses of health programs, see E. J. Mishan, "Evaluation of Life and Limb.: A Theoretical Approach," *Journal of Political Economy,* July-August 1971.

3. Such imperfections and an analysis of possible remedies are discussed in Milton Friedman's *Capitalism and Freedom,* Chapter 6, University of Chicago Press, Chicago, 1962; and Marc Nerlove, "On Tuition and the Costs of Higher Education: Prolegomena to a Conceptual Framework," *Journal of Political Economy,* Part II, May-June 1972.

4. M. Nerlove, op. cit., p. 5215.

5. For an excellent discussion of the use of auxiliaries in other countries, particularly New Zealand, and their effect on dental health status of the population, see Ruth Roemer, "The Legal Scope of Dental Hygienists in the United States and Other Countries," *Public Health Reports,* November 1970. Also see W. J. Pelton, H. Bethart, K. Goller, "The Ability of Dental Therapists to Perform Oral Prophylaxis," *Journal of the American Dental Association,* March 1972.

6. "Does Licensing Help?" *Consumer Reports,* February 1967, p. 110. The conclusion of an article on the quality of TV repair services concludes with the statement that "licensing boards that decry shady business practices without attempting to uncover them provide only the most limited consumer protection."

7. For some articles that are critical of the increasing movement toward licensure for health manpower, see, Nathan Hershey, "New Directions in Licensure of Health Personnel," *Economic and Business Bulletin,* Temple University, Fall 1971; and Rick J. Carlson, "Health Manpower Licensing and Emerging Institutional Responsibility for the Quality of Care," *Law and Contemporary Problems,* Part II, School of Law, Duke University, Autumn 1970.

8. There have been several articles and books on the medical profession in its use of restrictions as a means of limiting entry into the profession. See, for example, Reuben Kessel, "Price Discrimination in Medicine," *Journal of Law and Economics,* October 1958; Milton Friedman, "Occupational Licensure," in *Capitalism and Freedom,* University of Chicago Press, 1962; and Elton Rayack, *Professional Power and American Medicine: The Economics of the American Medical Association,* World Publishing Company, Cleveland, 1967.

9. Requirements for licensure that appear to be unrelated to quality are citizenship, minimum age, and minimum state residence. Also, all states require six years of professional education. *State Licensing of Health Occupations,* Public Health Service Publication, No. 1758, U.S. Department of Health, Education, and Welfare, National Center for Health Statistics, Washington, D.C., p. 45.

10. C. M. Lindsay, "Supply Response to Public Financing of Medical Care in the United States," Unpublished Doctoral Dissertation, University of Virginia, 1968.

11. There are three publications which are of particular interest with respect to restrictions in dentistry; the first is the *Reports of the Special Committees,* prepared for the Task Force on National Health Programs of the American Dental Association; the second is *A Report with Recommendations* which was in turn prepared by the Task Force for the Board of Trustees and the House of Delegates of the American Dental Association, and the last is the *Guidelines for Dentistry's Position in a National Health Program* which was adopted by the 1971 House of Delegates of the American Dental Association in October 1971.

There were many recommendations that were proposed in the initial reports by the Special Committees that were eventually adopted by both the Task Force and by the House of Delegates. Some of these were far reaching and innovative. However, a number of recommendations made by the Special Committees, particularly in the area of fewer restrictions on entry into the profesion, inter-state mobility, and on performance of tasks, were either modified, rejected or dropped or referred for further study, in the series of guidelines finally adopted by the House of Delegates.

12. W. Lee Hansen and B. A. Weisbrod, "The Distribution of Costs and Benefits of Public Higher Education: The Case of California," *Journal of Human Resources,* Spring 1969.

13. This proposition is demonstrated graphically in most texts on microeconomics, see for example, Donald S. Watson, *Price Theory and Its Uses* (2nd ed.), Houghton Mifflin Company, Boston, 1968, p. 96.

14. Paul Feldman, "Efficiency, Distribution, and the Role of Government in a Market Economy," *Journal of Political Economy,* May-June, 1971, pp. 524-252.

15. The discussion in this section is based upon Irv Garfinkel, *Financing Medical Care: A Welfare Economics Analysis,* Unpublished Doctoral Dissertation, University of Michigan, 1970.

Bibliography

Periodicals

American Dental Association, Bureau of Economic Research and Statistics "Inventory of Dentists – 1964," *Journal of the American Dental Association,* Vol. 70, May 1965, pp. 1261-1269.

American Dental Association, Bureau of Economic Research and Statistics, "Number of Dental Graduates Required Annually to 1985," *Journal of the American Dental Association,* Vol. 71, September 1969.

American Dental Association, Council on Dental Care Programs, "Dental Insurance is Different," *Journal of the American Dental Association,* Vol. 83, No. 4, October 1971, p. 754.

Ast, David B., et. al., "Time and Cost Factors to Provide Regular, Periodic Dental Care for Children in a Fluoridated and Non-Fluoridated Areas: Final Report," *Journal of the American Dental Association,* April, 1970.

Bethart, H.; Goller, K., and Pelton, W. J., "The Ability of Dental Therapists to Perform Oral Prophylaxis," *Journal of the American Dental Association,* March 1972.

Blayney, J. R., and Hill, I. N., "Flourine and Dental Caries," *Journal of the American Dental Association* (special issue), January 1967.

Brightman, I., and Allaway, N., "Evaluation of Medical and Dental Care Under the Medical Assistance Program," *American Journal of Public Health,* December 1969.

Carlson, Rick J., "Health Manpower Licensing and Emerging Institutional Responsibility for the Quality of Care," *Law and Contemporary Problems,* Part II, School of Law, Duke University, Autumn 1970.

Castaldi, C. R., "Dental Auxiliaries: Dentistry's Dilemma," *Journal of the American Dental Association,* May 1972.

Cole, Roger B., and Cohen, Lois K., "Dental Manpower: Estimating Resources and Requirements," *The Milbank Memorial Fund Quarterly,* Part 2, July 1971.

Douglas, Bruce L.; Wallace, Donald A.; Lerner, Monroe; and Coppersmith, Sylvia, "Impact of Water Fluoridation on Dental Practice and Dental Manpower," *Journal of the American Dental Association,* Vol. 84, February, 1972, pp. 355-367.

Feldman, Paul, "Efficiency, Distribution, and the Role of Government in a Market Economy," *Journal of Political Economy,* May/June 1971.

Feldstein, M. S., "The Use of An Econometric Model for Health Sector Planning," Discussion Paper No. 14, Cambridge: Harvard Institute for Economic Research, 1968.

Hansen, W. Lee, "Equity and the Finance of Higher Education," *Journal of Political Economy,* Vol. 80, No. 3, Part 2, May/June 1972.

Hansen, W. Lee, and Weisbrod, B. A., "The Distribution of Costs and Benefits of Public Higher Education: The Case of California," *Journal of Human Resources,* Spring 1969.

Hershey, Nathan, "New Directions in Licensure of Health Personnel," *Economic Business Bulletin,* Temple University, Fall 1971.

Holen, Arlene S., "Effects of Professional Licensing Arrangements on Interstate Labor Mobility and Resource Allocation," *Journal of Political Economy,* October 1965.

Jones, Robert C., "Dentist's View on Reimbursement Arrangements Under Prepayment and Insurance Plans," *Journal of the American Dental Association,* Vol. 84, No. 1, January 1972.

Jong, A., and Leske, G., "Utilization and Cost of Dental Services for Pre-School Children in Boston's Head Start Program," *Journal of Public Health Dentistry,* Spring 1968.

Kessel, Reuben, "Price Discrimination in Medicine," *Journal of Law and Economics,* October 1958.

Mason, Henry R., "Effectiveness of Student Aid Programs Tied to a Service Committment," *Journal of Medical Education,* July 1971.

Miller, Herman P., "Annual and Lifetime Income in Relation to Education: 1939-1959," *American Economic Review,* December 1960.

Mishan, E. J., "Evaluation of Life and Limb: A Theoretical Approach," *Journal of Political Economy,* July/August 1971.

Moen, Duane, and Poetsch, W. E., "More Preventive Care, Less Tooth Repair," *Journal of the American Dental Association,* Vol. 81, July 1970.

Morris, Alvin L. and Greulich, Richard C., "National Institute of Dental Research Inter-disciplinary Programs have Broadened the Base of Dental Science," *Science,* Vol. 160, June 7, 1968, pp. 1081-1088.

Nerlove, Marc, "On Tuition and the Costs of Higher Education: Prolegomena to a Conceptual Framework," *Journal of Political Economy,* Part II, May/June 1972.

Newhouse, Joseph, "The Economics of Group Practice," The Rand Corporation, 1971.

O'Shea, R. M.; Rosner, J. F.; Bissell, G. D.; and Johnston, D. W., "The Impact of Medicaid on Dental Practice: Some Evidence from Erie County, New York," *New York Dental Journal,* November 1969.

Pauly, Mark, "The Economics of Moral Hazard: Comment," *American Economic Review,* June 1968.

Riedel, Donald C., and Lerner, Monroe, "The Impact of Prepayment on the Economics of Dental Care," *Journal of the American Dental Association,* April 1966.

Roemer, Ruth, "The Legal Scope of Dental Hygienists in the United States and Other Countries," *Public Health Reports,* November 1970.

Ross, Blanche E., "A Comparative Study of Four Dental Payments Mechanisms in a Head Start Program," *American Journal of Public Health,* Vol. 61, Number 11, November, 1971, pp. 2176-2187.

Samuelson, Paul A., "The Pure Theory of Public Expenditure," *Review of Economics and Statistics,* November 1954.

Schultz, Theodore, "Capital Formation by Education," *Journal of Political Economy,* December 1960.

Soricelli, David A., "Practical Experience in Peer Review Controlling Quality in the Delivery of Dental Care," *American Journal of Public Health,* October 1971.

Upton, C., and Silverman, W., "The Demand for Dental Services," *The Journal of Human Resources,* Spring 1972.

Weinfeld, William, "Income of Dentists, 1928-1948," *Survey of Current Business* (U.S. Department of Commerce), January 1950.

Yett, Donald, "An Evaluation of Methods of Estimating Physician's Expenses Relative to Output," *Inquiry,* March 1967.

Zipporah, H., and Leatherwood, E., "A Dental Program for Head Start Children In New York City: A Retrospective Study of Utilization and Costs," *Medical Care,* July-August 1969.

"Does Licensing Help?" *Consumer Reports,* February 1967.

Announcements (for 1930, 1939-1940, 1951-1952, 1955-1956, 1960-1961), School of Dentistry, University of Michigan.

Fluoride Abstracts. Published periodically by Department of Environmental Health, Kettering Laboratory, College of Medicine, University of Cincinnati, Cincinnati, Ohio.

Books

American Association of Dental Schools, *Cost Study of Dental Education 1963-1964,* Chapel Hill, North Carolina, 1965.

American Council on Education, Commission on the Survey of Dentistry in the United States, *The Survey of Dentistry.* Washington, D.C.: American Council on Education, 1961.

Anderson, O. W.; Collette, P.; and Feldman, J. J., *Family Expenditure Patterns for Personal Health Services.* Health Information Foundation Research Series, No. 14.

Anderson, Robert, and Benham, Lee, "Factors Affecting the Relationship Between Family Income and Medical Care Consumption," in *Empirical Studies in Health Economics,* Ed. by H. Klarman. Baltimore: The Johns Hopkins University Press, 1970.

Bailey, Richard, "Economies of Scale in Medical Practice," in *Empirical Studies in Health Economics,* Ed. by H. Klarman. Baltimore: The Johns Hopkins University Press, 1970.

Buchanan, James M., *The Demand and Supply of Public Goods.* Chicago: Rand, McNally and Company, 1968.

Campbell, I. R., *Role of Fluoride in Public Health: The Soundness of Fluoridation in Communal Water Supplies, A Selected Bibliography.* Cincinnati: University of Cincinnati, 1963.

Dean, B. V.; Bhat, U. N.; Singh, A. J.; and Das, J., *Prepaid Dental Plan: Final Report.* Technical Memorandum No. 141, Cleveland: Operations Research Department, School of Management, Case Western Reserve University, 1969.

Feldstein, Paul J., "The Demand for Medical Care," in Report of the *Commission on the Cost of Medical Care,* American Medical Association, Vol. 1, 1964.

Feldstein, P. J., and Kelman, S., "An Econometric Model of the Medical Care Sector," in *Empirical Studies in Health Economics,* Ed. by H. Klarman. New York: Columbia University Press, 1970.

Friedman, Milton, *Capitalism and Freedom.* Chicago: University of Chicago Press, 1962.

Fusillo, Alice E., and Metz, A. Stafford, "Social Science Research on the Dental Student," in *Social Sciences and Dentistry: A Critical Bibliography.* Ed. by N. D. Richards and L. K. Cohen. The Hague, Netherlands: A. Sijthoff, 1971.

Hansen, W. Lee, "Shortages and Investment in Health Manpower," *The Economics of Health and Medical Care, Proceedings of the Conference on Economics of Health and Medical Care, May 10-12, 1962.* Ann Arbor: The University of Michigan, 1969.

Katona, George; Mandell, Lewis; and Schmideskamp, Jay, *1970 Survey of Consumer Finances.* Ann Arbor: Survey Research Center, Institute for Social Research, University of Michigan, 1971.

Leftwich, R. A., *The Price System and Resource Allocation.* New York: Holt, Reinhart, and Winston, 1970.

McClure, Frank J., *Water Fluoridation, the Search and the Victory.* National Institutes of Health, 1970.

Maurizi, Alex R., *Economic Essays on the Dental Profession.* Iowa City, Iowa: College of Business Administration, The University of Iowa, 1969.

Musgrave, Richard A., *The Theory of Public Finance.* New York: McGraw-Hill Book Company, 1959.

Newman, John F., and Anderson, Odin W., *Patterns of Dental Service Utilization in the United States: A Nationwide Survey* (Research Series 30). Chicago: Center for Health Administration Studies, University of Chicago, 1972.

Pelton, Walter T., and Bothwell, Ruth D., "The Need and The Demand for Dental Care," in *Proceedings of the Workshop on Future Requirements on*

Dental Manpower and the Training and Utilization of Auxiliary Personnel. Ann Arbor: University of Michigan, 1972.

Rayak, Elton, *Professional Power and American Medicine: The Economics of the American Medical Association.* Cleveland: World Publishing Company, 1967.

Richards, N. David, "Utilization of Dental Services," in *Social Sciences and Dentistry: A Critical Bibliography.* The Hague, Netherlands: A. Sijthoff, 1971.

Tax Foundation, Inc., *Facts and Figures on Government Finance,* 13th ed. New York. 1964-1965.

Watson, Donald S., *Price Theory and Its Uses,* 2nd ed. New York: Houghton Mifflin Company, 1968.

Young, W., and Striffler, D., *The Dentist, His Practice, His Community,* 2nd ed. Philadelphia: W. B. Saunders Company, 1969.

Fluorides and Human Health. World Health Organization Monograph #59, 1970.

Report of the Royal Commissioner into the Fluoridation of Public Water Supplies, Tasmania, 1968.

Royal Commission on Health Services, Vol. 1, Ottowa, Canada: Queen's Printer, 1964.

American Dental Association Publications

American Dental Association, *The Annual Report on Dental Education 1970-1971: Financial Information,* Chicago, 1971.

American Dental Association, *Distribution of Dentists in the United States by state, region, district and county,* 1970.

American Dental Association, *Survey of Dental Practice* (for 1950, 1953, 1956, 1959, 1962, 1965, 1968), 1971.

American Dental Association, Council on Dental Education, *Annual Report on Dental Auxiliary Education,* 1967-1968, 1968-1969, 1969-1970.

American Dental Association, Task Force on National Health Programs, "The Requirements for Dental and Dental Auxiliary Manpower," *Dentistry in National Health Programs: Reports of the Special Committees,* Chicago, 1971.

American Dental Association, Task Force on National Health Programs, *Dentistry in National Health Programs.* A Report with Recommendations. *Journal of the American Dental Association,* September 1971.

Guidelines for Dentistry's Position in a National Health Program, adopted by the 1971 House of Delegates of the American Dental Association, October 1971,

The Journal of the American Dental Association, Vol. 83, No. 6, December 1971.

Moen, Duane B.; Ogawa, George Y.; and Denne, John D., *Survey of Needs for Dental Care, 1965,* American Dental Association, Chicago, November, 1966.

Unpublished Papers

Garfinkel, Irv, "Financing Medical Care: A Welfare Economics Analysis," unpublished Ph.D. dissertation, University of Michigan, 1970.

Lindsay, C. M., "Supply Response to Public Financing of Medical Care in the United States," unpublished Ph.D. dissertation, University of Virginia, 1968.

Newman, John F., Jr., "The Utilization of Dental Services," unpublished Ph.D. dissertation, Emory University, 1971.

Weiss, Jeffrey, "The Changing Job Structure of Health Manpower," unpublished Ph.D. dissertation, Harvard University, 1966.

Unpublished Data and Correspondence

Correspondence with Ruth Bothwell, Division of Dental Health, Public Health Service, Department of Health, Education, and Welfare.

American Dental Association, Council on Dental Education, Applicants to Dental School in 1967 and previous years.

American Dental Association, Council on Dental Education, Unpublished data from Dental Students' Register Questionnaire for 1961-1962, and Dental Students' Register, 1959-1960, through 1966-1967.

American Dental Association, Council on Dental Education, Correspondence with James A. Mastio, Project Director, Annual Report on Dental Education.

Data from the Bureau of Research and Statistics, American Dental Association, 1970.

Data from the Health Interview Survey, National Center for Health Statistics, Public Health Service, Department of Health, Education, and Welfare, Rockville, Maryland.

University of Michigan Placement Service, from College Placement Council, *Salary Survey,* July 1971.

Government Publications

Bureau of Health Manpower Education, Division of Manpower Intelligence, *Projections of Manpower Resources in Selected Health Professions,*

1970-1980, Report No. 72-58, Washington, D.C.: Government Printing Office, February 1972.

U.S. Bureau of Census, "Educational Attainment by Economic Characteristics," in *1940 Census of Population, Education*, Washington, D.C.: Government Printing Office, 1940.

U.S. Bureau of Census, *1950 Census of the Population: Series P.E., No. 5B Education*, Washington, D.C.: Government Printing Office, 1950.

U.S. Bureau of Census, *Current Population Survey* (Consumer Income Supplement). Washington, D.C.: Government Printing Office, 1947, 1959, 1964.

U.S. Bureau of Census, *Current Population Survey* (Series P-25, Nos. 304 – April 8, 1965; 348 – September 16, 1966; 414 – January 28, 1969), Washington, D.C.: Government Printing Office.

U.S. Bureau of Census, *Statistical Abstract of the United States*, Washington, D.C.: Government Printing Office, 1950-1971.

U.S. Bureau of the Census, *U.S. Historical Statistics*, Washington, D.C.: Government Printing Office, Colonial Times to 1957, and 1962 Supplement for 1930-1960.

Cooper, Barbara S., *National Health Expenditures, 1929-1967*, Social Security Administration, Office of Research and Statistics, Research and Statistics Note No. 16, September 29, 1969.

Cooper, Barbara, and McGee, Mary, *National Health Expenditures, Fiscal Years 1929-1970 and Calendar Years 1929-1969*, Social Security Administration, Office of Research and Statistics, Research and Statistics Note No. 25, December 14, 1970.

Cooper, Barbara S., and Worthington, Nancy L., *National Health Expenditures, Calendar Years 1929-1970*. Social Security Administration, Office of Research and Statistics, Research and Statistics Note No. 1, January 14, 1972.

Hanft, Ruth S., *National Health Expenditures by Object of Expenditures and Source of Funds, 1950-1963*, Social Security Administration, Office of Research and Statistics, Research and Statistics Note No. 6, April 5, 1966.

Rice, Dorothy P., and Cooper, Barbara S., "National Health Expenditures 1950-1966," *Social Security Bulletin*, April, 1968.

U.S. Congress. House. Committee on Interstate and Foreign Commerce. *Hearings* on H.R. 703, 4171, 4155, 5614, 5767, 7765, 4145, 4156, 4618, 7707, 7736 before the subcommittee on Public Health and Environment: Statement of Dr. James Bowden, Dean, University of North Carolina School of Dentistry, in behalf of the American Dental Association and American Association of Dental Schools; accompanied by Dr. Richard K. Mosbaugh, Chairman, Council on Legislation, ADA, and Hal M. Christensen, Director, Washington Office, ADA 92nd Congress, 1st sess., April 2, 3, 20, 21, 22, 27, 28, 29, 1971.

254

U.S. Congress. House. Committee on Interstate and Foreign Commerce. *Hearings* on H.R. 4999, 8774, and 8833, Statement of Honorable Abraham Ribicoff, Secretary, accompanied by Wilbur J. Cohen, Assistant Secretary, Boisfeuillet Jones, Special Assistant to the Secretary, Health and Medical Affairs, and Dr. Luther L. Terry, Surgeon General, Public Health Service, Department of Health, Education and Welfare. Washington, D.C.: Government Printing Office, January, 1962.

U.S. Congress. House. Committee on Interstate and Foreign Commerce. *Hearings* on H.R. 4999, 8774, 8833, Summary Statement of the American Dental Association. Washington, D.C.: Government Printing Office, January 1962, p. 178.

U.S. Congress. Senate. Committee on Labor and Public Welfare. *Hearings* on S.595 and H.R. 3141, Prepared Statement of the American Association of Dental Schools. Washington, D.C.: Government Printing Office, September 1965.

U.S. Congress. Senate. Committee on Labor and Public Welfare. *Hearings* on S.595 and H.R. 3141, Prepared Statement of David A. Bensinger, D.D.S., Assistant Dean, Washington University, School of Dentistry, St. Louis, Mo. Washington, D.C.: Government Printing Office, 1970.

U.S. Congress. Senate. Committee on Labor and Public Welfare. *Hearings* before the Subcommittee on Health on S.595 and H.R. 3141, Statement of Dr. Maynard K. Hine, President-Elect, Dean, School of Dentistry, Indiana University; Accompanied by Dr. A. Ray Baralt, Jr., Dean, School of Dentistry, University of Detroit; Dr. Reginald H. Sullens, Executive Secretary, American Association of Dental Schools; and Mr. Hal M. Christensen, Director of the Washington Office, American Dental Association. Washington, D.C.: Government Printing Office, September 1965.

U.S. Congress. Senate. Committee on Labor and Public Welfare. *Hearings* before the Subcommittee on Health on S.911 and H.R. 12. Statment of Boisfeuillet Jones, Special Assistant for Health and Medical Affairs, U.S. Department of Health, Education, and Welfare, accompanied by Dr. Luther Terry, Surgeon General, U.S. Public Health Service. Washington, D.C.: Government Printing Office, August 22, 23, 26, 1963, p. 69.

U.S. Congress. Senate, Committee on Labor and Public Welfare. *Report on S.934, July 12, 1971.* Washington, D.C.: Government Printing Office, July 1971.

U.S. Department of Health, Education, and Welfare. *Fluoridated Drinking Waters* Ed. by F. J. McClure. Washington, D.C.: Government Printing Office, 1962.

U.S. Department of Health, Education, and Welfare, Division of Dental Health. *Fluoridation Saves Teeth, Dollars, and Dental Manpower.* Washington, D.C.: Government Printing Office, August, 1971.

U.S. Department of Health, Education, and Welfare, National Institutes of Health. *Fluoride Census.* Washington, D.C.: Government Printing Office, 1965-1969.

U.S. Department of Health, Education, and Welfare, Public Health Service. *Fluoride Drinking Waters.* Washington, D.C.: Government Printing Office, 1962.

Pelton, Walter J.; Pennell, Elliot H.; and Vaura, Helen, M., *Health Manpower Source Book – Dental Hygienists.* Public Health Service Publication No. 263, Section 8. Washington, D.C.: Government Printing Office, 1957.

U.S. Department of Health, Education, and Welfare, *Health Manpower Source Book: Section 20, Manpower Supply and Educational Statistics;* Manpower Studies Branch, Division of Dental Health, Public Health Service, Washington, D.C.: Government Printing Office, updated to March 1971.

U.S. Department of Health, Education, and Welfare. *The Health Professions Educational Assistance Program: Report to the President and Congress,* Washington, D.C.: Government Printing Office, September 1970.

U.S. Department of Health, Education, and Welfare. *How Medical Students Finance Their Education,* by Louis C. R. Smith and Anna R. Crocker. Public Health Service Publication No. 1336-1, Washington, D.C.: Government Printing Office, 1970, p. 8.

U.S. Department of Health, Education, and Welfare. "The Development of a Micro-Simulation Model of Health Manpower Demand and Supply," by D. E. Yett; L. Drabek; M.D. Intrilligator; and L. J. Kimball in *Proceedings and Report of Conference on a Health Manpower Simulation Model,* Washington, D.C.: Government Printing Office, 1970.

U.S. Department of Health, Education, and Welfare. *State Licensing of Health Occupations,* Public Health Service Publication, No. 1758. Washington, D.C.: Government Printing Office, p. 45.

U.S. Department of Health, Education, and Welfare. *Health Statistics from the U.S. National Health Survey: Dental Care, Volume of Visits, United States, July 1957-June 1959,* Series B-No. 15, Washington, D.C.: Government Printing Office, April 1960, pp. 12-13.

U.S. Department of Health, Education, and Welfare, Public Health Service, *Monthly Vital Statistics Report: Health-Interview Survey-Provisional Data from the National Center for Health Statistics,* Vol. 18, No. 9, Supplement 2, Washington, D.C.: Government Printing Office, December 18, No. 9, pp. 4-5.

U.S. Department of Health, Education, and Welfare, *Volume of Dental Visits, United States, July 1963-June 1964,* Public Health Service Publication No. 1000 – Series 10, No. 23, Washington, D.C.: Government Printing Office, October 1965, pp. 17-18.

U.S. Department of Justice, Immigration and Naturalization Service, *Annual Reports,* Washington, D.C.: Government Printing Office, 1959-1970.

U.S. Department of Labor, Bureau of Labor Statistics, *Monthly Labor Review.* Washington, D.C.: Government Printing Office.

Water Fluoridation Practices in Major Cities in the United States. A report prepared for the New York State Department of Health by the New York University College of Engineering, p. 54, Table 15.

Index

ADA, *see* American Dental Association
Age-visit ratios, 31, 51, 200
Alabama, 97
American Dental Association (ADA): 25,
  64, 75–76, 77n., 116, 126, 129, 130;
  Bureau of Membership and Records, 64;
  Council on Dental Education, 134;
  House of Delegates, 244–45: surveys
  and data, 23, 75–77, 80, 131, 143, 185
Arkansas, 97
Attitudes toward dental care: 28–29, 34;
  and education, 51, 182
Auxiliaries: 12, 61, 70, 72–73, 83–85, 163;
  education, 105–12, 133, 235; licensing,
  107, 188–89, 221, 234; part-time, 74n.;
  productivity, 63, 70, 72, 78–80, 82–83,
  84, 88–133, 143, 167; restrictions on
  use, 221, 222; wages, 17, 68, 78, 85–87,
  88, 107, 193, 243

Bane report, 129–30
Benham, Lee, 58
Berry, Ralph E., xvii
Brown, Dr. William, xvii
Bureau of Census, 241
Bureau of Health Manpower Education,
  242
Bureau of Labor Statistics, 75–78

Canadian dentists, 65–66
Capitation, 13, 43, 115–16
Census of Population, 65
Coinsurance, 46–49, 197–98, 205, 206,
  230
Complementary health care programs, 3
"Composite Fee" (ADA), 72, 77n.
Construction costs, 13, 96, 117, 127
Consumer Expenditure Survey, 76n., 77n.
Consumer Price Index, 25
Copayments: 29, 40, 45, 46; and
  coinsurance, 49
Corporate dental practice, 24n.
Cost-benefit analysis, 179–80
Current Population Reports, 240

Deductibles, 29, 42, 45–46, 197–98, 205,
  206
Demand: 7–8, 27–40; and dental insurance,
  45–49; and income, 54, 59, 143, 152,
  165, 229; and population, 59, 142, 149
Dental assistants: 105, 110, 111, 234, 235;
  see also Auxiliaries
Dental Care Price Index, 75
Dental graduates, 13, 97, 166, 224n., 241,
  242

Dental hygienist: 105, 111, 235; *see also*
  Auxiliaries
Dental insurance: 29, 37, 40–50; actuarial
  costs, 40–41, 42; administrative costs,
  41; and demand, 41–50, 52; and family
  income, 42, 46, 50; premiums, 45;
  see also National dental insurance plan
Dental manpower: 5, 12, 13, 154–59, 242;
  and dental school space, 145
Dental students: 7; costs, 7, 121; family
  income, 120, 236; quality, 106–107;
  see also Scholarships and loans
Dental technicians: 105, 111, 112, 235;
  see also Auxiliaries
Dentist-population ratio, 12, 19, 64, 231
Dentist schools: 13–15, 17, 51, 58, 90,
  95–98, 187; applicants, 7, 106; auxiliaries, 12, 15n., 133; construction, 96,
  117, 123–25, 155; enrollments, 13,
  133, 237, 238; spaces, 15, 123; and sub-
  sidies, 60, 92, 106, 117, 125–26, 133–34
Department of Health, Education and Welfare, 23, 34, 127, 149; Division of
  Dental Health, 64, 65, 126, 242
Determinants of demand, 7, 28–40
Determinants of supply, 62–67
Distribution of dental service, 60–61
Distribution of Dentists (ADA), 64–65,
  130, 240
Division of Manpower Intelligence, 242

Econometric model: 18–19, 141–74; and
  forecasts, 147–53; and policy analysis,
  153–66; and ratio technique, 148–53,
  166
Economies of scale, 60, 108, 112–16,
  135–39
Education: 36, 92–93, 105; and attitudes
  to dental work, 51, 182
Equity objectives: 220; *see also* Income redistribution
Examinations, 31, 37
Expenditures on oral health: 2–3, 12, 19,
  20–27, 39, 50–51, 76–79, 146; forecasts, 21, 27; and income, 23, 37, 40;
  1940–1970, 22; per capita, 23–27, 46,
  51; and supply, 61–62, 73–78

Federal funds: 1, 5, 12, 87, 116–18, 175–
  207, 222; *see also* Health Professions
  Education Act *and* Subsidies
Fee-for-service, 43, 44
Fees, 75–78
Fillings, 31, 37, 76n., 77n.
Florida, 97

257

About The Author

Paul J. Feldstein received the Ph.D. in 1961 from the University of Chicago, where he was the first W. K. Kellogg Fellow. It was while he was looking for a dissertation topic that he became interested in the economics of health. He then served as Director of the Division of Research at the American Hospital Association, where he started the monthly HOSPITAL INDICATORS survey. He has been at the University of Michigan since 1964, where he is currently Professor in the Program in Hospital Administration at the School of Public Health and has a joint appointment in the Department of Economics.

In 1967-1968, while Professor Feldstein was on leave of absence from the University, he served at the Bureau of the Budget and the Social Security Administration in Washington. He spent 1972-1973 as an economic consultant to the World Health Organization in Geneva. The author is a consultant to the Department of Health, Education, and Welfare and other health organizations. His previous research and writings have been on the economics of medical care.